MEDICAL TERMINOLOGY FOR EVERYONE

MEDICAL TERMINOLOGY FOR EVERYONE

Easily Learn, Memorize, and Pronounce Medical Terms

John Louis Temple, MD

ROCKRIDGE
PRESS

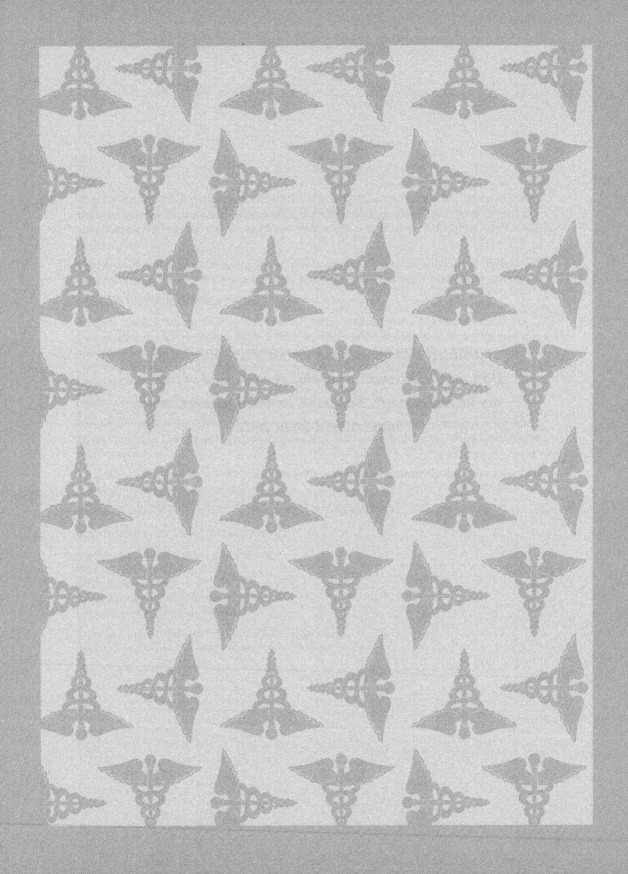

CONTENTS

INTRODUCTION ix

HOW TO USE THIS BOOK xi

PART I: MEDICAL AND ANATOMICAL TERMINOLOGY 1

    CHAPTER 1: Understanding Medical Terms 3

    CHAPTER 2: How the Body Is Organized 19

PART II: MEDICAL TERMS BY ROOT, PREFIX, AND SUFFIX 37

    CHAPTER 3: Root Words of the Body's Systems 39

    CHAPTER 4: Root Words for Internal and
             External Body Parts 65

    CHAPTER 5: Prefixes 79

    CHAPTER 6: Suffixes 99

    CHAPTER 7: Homophones, Eponyms, Acronyms,
             Abbreviations, and Symbols 117

A FINAL NOTE 134

RESOURCES 136

REFERENCES 139

INDEX 140

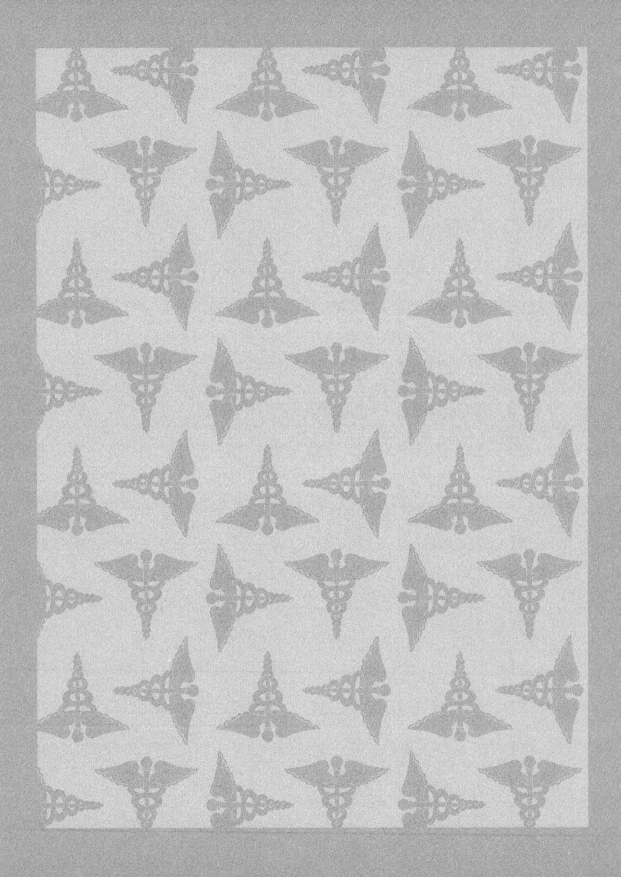

INTRODUCTION

Hello and welcome! My name is John Temple, and I am an internal medicine physician practicing in Southern California. I specialize in hospital medicine, which means I treat adults with a wide variety of conditions, including infections, diabetic complications, liver disease, heart attacks, and much more. One of the best aspects of internal medicine is the sheer diversity of conditions we see.

In case you are unfamiliar with the medical training process: I completed a bachelor's degree in biology, four years of medical school, three years of internal medicine residency, and one year as an internal medicine chief resident. I am now going on my fourth year as a fully independent attending physician. It has been quite the journey, and each step has brought its fair share of enjoyment and challenges. I would do it all again, and I highly encourage anyone planning to pursue medicine to take the journey as well.

I wrote this book with one simple goal in mind: to improve communication between health-care providers and patients. All too often, physicians use medical jargon that leaves patients confused, scared, and vulnerable. When providers have a more comprehensive understanding of the terminology, they can more easily explain the meaning to patients. When patients have a baseline understanding of medical terms, they are empowered to ask informed questions about their care and conditions. Ultimately, improving this communication serves to better connect all of us, which leads to better health care. I hope that you will someday become an expert on navigating both languages.

Since anatomy and physiology classes, early in my undergraduate training, I have been fascinated by medical terminology. To an outsider, the words may seem complex and cryptic, often with a poetic quality about them. I actually find them very descriptive and specific. The secret is that medical terms are not terribly complicated. In fact, if you know Greek and Latin, the terms are quite basic. For example, the term "hydrophobia" is Greek for "water-scared," or a fear of water. I recommend that you try to link the terminology throughout this book to anatomy, diseases, and other words that you already recognize. Try to find elements within words that resemble English words. With a little imagination, you can see how many elements of medical terminology are found in daily life. Of course, any foreign language is challenging at first, but by the end of this book, you will be confident in your ability to understand and use medical terminology whether you are a patient or a provider.

HOW TO USE THIS BOOK

This book is not a dictionary or an encyclopedia. It does not contain every single medical term ever coined. A book like that would take up an entire room. This book is small enough to carry and contains the most important medical terminology I use on a daily basis as a clinician. It will provide you with a framework to quickly decode and understand nearly every medical term, as well as real-world examples to help you retain the information. It will also occasionally explain how the roots of medical terms can be found in non-medical terms that we use in our daily lives.

This book is intentionally structured to lay a strong foundation of knowledge from which to build. I recommend reading this book from start to finish. You can then refer to specific sections as you advance in your training. Feel free to make notes, underline, highlight, and "dog-ear" pages. We will later discuss how to best study this material, but I prefer to make the tables into flash cards for efficient memorization. Each chapter concludes with a quiz that will allow you to test your knowledge. During my training, I took countless quizzes and tests because I always find they help me better retain information.

Finally, I want to let you in on a little secret: Putting on a crisp, clean white coat makes a doctor feel a little more confident and competent. When you have this book at your side, I hope you feel the same.

pan stasis physis
ipsi septo intus
tort ileo hepat
intra chondro pe
neuro cyte vas
deno ular ca
chole itis sarco ta
rectomy cephalo
edema esis trophy
sarcoma osis
pseudo xeno le
oxy thorac hydr
andr cili ren
cepha

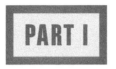

MEDICAL AND ANATOMICAL TERMINOLOGY

To learn, understand, and memorize anything (especially a new language), it is important to start with a strong foundation. Part 1 of this book gives you just that. You will learn why it is essential for everybody, not just people who work in health care, to understand medical terminology. Then I will share my favorite way to study and memorize this material. I understand your time is precious, so I will give you my top tips for efficiency.

You will then learn how to break down medical terms into their component pieces. Most medical terms are created by combining smaller words or components. When you know how to tease apart terms, you can see an unfamiliar word for the first time, dissect it, and make a highly educated guess about its meaning. Even as a seasoned clinician, I occasionally run into new words and use this method to understand their meaning.

We will take a brief diversion into the ancient Greek and Latin origins of medical terminology. This is important because it helps you better understand how these words came to exist. Chapter 1 wraps up with rules that explain how to convert medical terms from singular to plural. Chapter 2 outlines the body's basic anatomical planes, positions, and cavities. This will provide a solid framework before we cover the organ systems in the subsequent chapters.

WHAT IS MEDICAL TERMINOLOGY?

Medical terminology is the language that health-care providers, as well scientists and researchers, use to communicate. It describes all the words and phrases used in health care and the basic health sciences. You may think of it as "doctor talk," but it spans many disciplines, including biology, anatomy, physiology, pathophysiology, histology, pharmacology, and microbiology. As we will discuss, the terms and their use have origins in Ancient Greek and Latin. Perhaps most important, medical terminology is often quite descriptive and precise, which is why it is the standard in today's health-care system. It allows those who use it to communicate clearly with each other. Whether one is conducting scientific research or diagnosing and treating an ailment, clear communication is vital.

There are medical terms for every cell, tissue, organ, organ system, and body part. There are terms that describe anatomical location, body position, size, shape, color, and texture. Medical terminology is more than just a collection of vocabulary terms. It truly is a language unto itself.

Later in this chapter, we will discuss how terms are actually built of subunits called prefixes, roots, and suffixes. These components can be arranged in a nearly infinite number of ways to create terms. You could create an entirely new term with these subunits, and a seasoned clinician would likely understand what you mean. How cool is that?

WHY LEARN MEDICAL TERMINOLOGY?

Medical terminology is like a foreign language. Whether we are wearing the white coat or speaking with someone who is, understanding the fundamentals of medical terminology is essential. Sometimes health-care providers use medical terms assuming everyone knows what they mean. I remember telling a patient they had "hypertension," only to be met with a very puzzled expression. I replied, "Oh, I'm sorry. I mean high blood pressure." As a patient, once you develop a foundational knowledge of medical terms, you will be able to better understand your body, medical conditions, procedures, and patient instructions. You will also be able to ask your medical team more specific questions.

And if you work, or plan to work, in health care, it is vital to be able to fluently speak this language. Medicine calls for precision in examination, imaging, lab work, diagnosis, and language. Learning medical terminology allows you to communicate information quickly and accurately with your team and ultimately allows you to provide high-quality care. I must admit that we, as clinicians, can do a better job speaking in a way that is understood by our patients. Once you complete this book, you will have solid footing in the medical language. I challenge you to then explain medical terms to someone outside of medicine to truly test your skills.

HOW TO STUDY AND MEMORIZE MEDICAL TERMINOLOGY

Everybody has their own way of learning and memorizing. Some people are visual learners, others are auditory learners, and some are kinesthetic, or hands-on, learners. This book can be used with whatever approach you prefer. For those who prefer visual learning, I find flash cards are the most efficient way to drill a large amount of information. I recommend putting the term and pronunciation on the front of the card and the meaning and an example on the back. For those who prefer auditory learning, some online flash card applications will read aloud to you. You can also practice with a partner. If you are a kinesthetic learner, you may find it especially useful to study these terms with a partner; use flash cards to quiz each other while standing, moving, and interacting.

I am typically an auditory and kinesthetic learner, but when I learned medical terminology, flash cards worked best for me. When I approach a stack of flash cards, I set aside the ones I know immediately, and I don't spend time on them. Then I focus my energy on the terms I'm unsure of or have no clue about. This allows me to whittle down the stack until I make it through all of the terms.

If you plan to use flash cards, you can use an app or a website, but studies have shown that words are better retained when handwritten. The hypothesis is that the movements of your hand and the tactile feedback help imprint memories in your brain. Even so, it takes time to scribble on both sides of a card; your pen can bleed through the paper, rendering the flash cards essentially useless; you need to remember to bring them with you to study; and in my case, I often spill coffee on them. So, if you prefer digital flash cards, I understand. There are many wonderful websites and mobile flash card applications. Quizlet (www.quizlet.com) is free, easy to navigate, and available in both a website and a mobile application. Other options to consider include Anki, Flashcards Maker, and Chegg.

I recommend making sets of flash cards for each of the tables in this book so that you can focus your study on a particular topic. You can study alone, but studying with others is usually more fun, and saying terms aloud to each other can help enhance memory.

To help you assess your progress, you'll find quizzes at the end of every chapter. You can write your answers directly in the book or, even better, use a piece of scratch paper for your answers so that you can quiz yourself again.

BREAKING MEDICAL TERMS APART

Nearly all medical terms can be broken into a prefix, root word, and suffix. Often you will find medical terms that are "prefix + root" or "root + suffix," and occasionally you will find complex words with "prefix + root + suffix." Occasionally, a root word can stand alone, such as the word "cell." However, neither a prefix nor a suffix can stand alone as a word.

I like to think of a medical term as a series of building blocks stuck together. Exchanging any of the blocks entirely changes the word's meaning. For instance, *hypo*thermia means something or someone is too cold. *Hyper*thermia is too hot. *Hypo*tension means blood pressure is too low, and *hyper*tension means that it is too high.

As you can imagine, there are nearly infinite ways to arrange the building blocks of words. By learning the foundational prefixes, root words, and suffixes, you will be able to understand exponentially more words than the ones contained in this book. You will even be able to create words of your own that have specific meaning, even if the words are not commonly used.

Listing every single medical term in this book would be both impractical and unnecessary. Understanding the meaning of medical prefixes, root words, and suffixes provides you the keys to unlock the meaning of an incredible number of medical terms. Just as you don't learn to speak French by memorizing every word in a French dictionary, you'll learn the language of medical terminology by understanding the rules behind the language. That said, you will encounter a vast amount of new medical terms along the way. Don't let unfamiliar words throw you; by the time you've finished reading this book, you'll be able to decipher nearly any medical term the first time you see it.

Prefix

A prefix is a letter, or the first few letters, of a word that shapes the word's meaning. The word "pre" is a Latin term that means "before" or "prior to." For example, think of the "previews" you watch before a movie. A prefix sets the tone for the word. Changing the prefix changes the word's meaning completely. Prefixes often describe color, amount, size, direction, or desirability (good or bad). Many prefixes may be familiar to you. For example, "trans" means "across," as in "*trans*portation," and "bi" means "two," as in *bi*cycle. We will dive deeply into prefixes in part 2 of this book.

Root

The "root word" is the core element of a medical term. It often relates to tissues, organs, organ systems, or disease processes. A word's root provides context and meaning. In rare cases, it can even stand alone without a prefix or suffix. Often, health-care providers use standalone root words informally when communicating. We often use the terms "neuro," "cardio," and "pulm" when discussing organ systems. Occasionally, medical terms will combine root words such as "cardiorenal," which refers to a process involving both the heart and the kidneys, or "gastrointestinal," which refers to the stomach ("gastro") and intestines.

Suffix

The word "suffix" comes from the Latin "suffixum," which essentially means "to attach below" or "to attach to the end." The suffix follows the root word and comprises the last few letters of a term. Much like the prefix, changing a suffix can dramatically affect the meaning of a word. One suffix that you will see a lot in this book is "-itis," meaning "inflammation." Another is "-oma," which means "mass." One of my favorite medical study tools is called

Pathoma, which literally means "a mass of pathology knowledge." Like a prefix, a suffix transforms the meaning of a word, so mastering suffixes is critical to understanding the medical language.

Example

An example of a medical term with a clear prefix, root word, and suffix is "atherosclerosis" (pronounced ATH-err-o-SKLER-oh-sis). "Athero" refers to arteries, "sclero" means "to harden," and "sis" refers to a process or condition. Thus, "atherosclerosis" means "the condition of hardened arteries." Another good example is "leukocytosis." The prefix "leuko" means "white," the root "cyte" means "cell," and the suffix "osis" means process or condition. A leukocytosis is when the white blood cells are elevated in the bloodstream, often indicating an ongoing infection or inflammatory state.

HOW TO COMBINE PREFIXES, ROOTS, AND SUFFIXES INTO WORDS

Even though we have not yet learned the common prefixes, root words, and suffixes, let's practice breaking medical terms into their components. We will begin with terms that may already be familiar to you.

Erythrocyte (eh-RITH-row-site): This term has a prefix, "erythro" (the color red), and root, "cyte" (a cell). Thus, the word "erythrocyte" means "red cell" and refers to red blood cells.

Neurology (nurr-AH-lo-gee): This term has a root, "neuro" (relating to the nervous system), and a suffix, "logy" ("the study of"). Thus, neurology is the study of the nervous system and its diseases.

Electrocardiogram (eh-leck-tro-CAR-dee-oh-gram): Often referred to as an "ECG," this term has all three elements: a prefix, "electro" (meaning "electrical"); a root word, "cardio" (meaning "heart"); and a suffix, "gram" (meaning "documentation" or "what is written"). Thus, an electrocardiogram is an electrical recording of the heart.

Now try to build your own medical term. Try to create a word that means "within the blood vessels." (Hint: Catheters that are placed in blood vessels are called IVs.) To assemble this term, we'll use the following parts:

The prefix for "within": intra-

The root word for "blood vessel": vasc

A suffix meaning "in relation to": -ular

Add that all together and you get "intravascular," often abbreviated as "IV." (We'll review common medical abbreviations in chapter 7.) If only putting in an IV were that easy.

There are a few important rules to be aware of when combining prefixes, roots, and suffixes. When combining a prefix and root, if the prefix ends in a vowel and the root word begins with a vowel, the prefix drops the ending letter.

EXAMPLE: Oligo + emia = Oligemia. This is a term that refers to diminished blood vessel marking seen on imaging, often in lung disease.

When combining a prefix and root or combining two root words, if the second word begins with a consonant, an "o" is added to the end of the first word.

EXAMPLES: cardiopulmonary, musculoskeletal, and sternoclavicular

I like to think of "o" as the glue that holds some of these building blocks together. These rules will become clearer as we go along. You will see terms listed with and without the trailing "o."

HOW TO PRONOUNCE MEDICAL TERMS

Learning the proper pronunciation of medical terms can be challenging, but it is critical for seamless communication. Ultimately, you must practice a term until you get it right. Many medical terms are long and, to the untrained eye, difficult to break into pronounceable pieces. However, as you now know, these lengthy terms are just a series of building blocks. If you know how to pronounce each block, then you can fairly accurately pronounce the entire word.

As with any language, medical terminology has a few distinct pronunciation conventions. Certain letters are silent, while others are pronounced in a distinct manner. Here is a list, in alphabetical order, of some common special pronunciations of which to be aware:

Ce sounds like "s," as in "cephalo" (pronounced "SEFF-a-low"); this relates to the head.

Cho sounds like "koll," as in "chole" (pronounced "KOLL-ee"); this relates to the gallbladder. The "h" is silent.

Cu sounds like "k," as in "cubit" (pronounced "KYOO-bit"); this relates to the elbow.

Ge sounds like "j," as in "geriatric" (pronounced "jer-ee-AA-trick"); this relates to the elderly.

Gyn sound like "guyn," as in "gynecology" (pronounced "GUY-neh-ko-lo-gy"); this relates to the female reproductive system.

Ph sounds like "f," as in "physio" (pronounced "FIH-zee-oh"); this relates to the body.

Pn sounds like "n" with a silent "p," as in "pneumo" (pronounced "NEW-mo"); this relates to the lungs.

Ps sounds like "s" with a silent "p," as in "pseudo" (pronounced "SOO-doh"); this relates to the term "false."

Pter sounds like "ter," as in "pterygium" (pronounced "ter-ih-GEE-um"); this relates to a wing-like growth of the cornea.

Rheu sounds like "roo," as in "rheum" (pronounced "room"); this relates to joints.

Xero sounds like "zero"; "xero" relates to the term "dry."

HOW TO USE THE PRONUNCIATION GUIDES IN THIS BOOK

Correct pronunciation of medical terminology is essential for accurate and effective communication. I deliberately chose to not use complex pronunciation systems, such as the International Phonetic Alphabet (IPA), because learning how to use that system is a formidable challenge. I want you to spend your valuable time learning medical terminology, not a phonetic alphabet, so I've provided the pronunciations that reflect the way that I, a seasoned clinician, would say each word.

Each term in this book is accompanied by a phonetic pronunciation guide. Each word is broken into syllables, and the syllables that have emphasis are in capital letters.

Here are a few examples:

Cholecystectomy: "KOLL-ee-sis-TEK-tuh-me"

Arthrocentesis: "arth-row-cent-EE-sis"

Pneumoperitoneum: "new-mo-per-ih-to-NEE-um"

CLASSICAL ORIGINS OF MEDICAL TERMINOLOGY

The origins of medical terminology are fascinating and could easily be an entire book in itself. Greek and Latin are the dominant ancestries; however, many languages have contributed, including Arabic, French, German, Spanish, Danish, and English.

Hippocrates, the famous Greek physician best known for authoring the Hippocratic Oath " . . . first do no harm," is considered the father of formal medical terminology. He documented the first terms in the 4th and 5th centuries BCE, more than 2400 years ago. An example of an Ancient Greek term still used today is "dyspnea," which means "bad or difficult breathing" and is a common term for shortness of breath. Another example is "cathar," which means "to flow out" and describes body contents flowing out of the digestive or genitourinary tracts. (This is the same origin as the word "catharsis," which is commonly used to describe the release of pent-up emotions or feelings.)

In the subsequent centuries, the Romans dominated Western Europe, and Latin became the dominant language. As a result, nearly every Greek medical term was modified and incorporated into Latin. Many countries around the world used Latin medical terms; however, as of the 1800s, native-language terms have become increasingly common.

Many medical terms were derived from animals, plants, and everyday objects. My favorite examples are the smallest bones in the body, the inner ear bones, known as the *malleus*, *incus*, and *stapes* because they resemble a "hammer," "anvil," and "stirrup," respectively. In the next few sections, we will dig deeper into these origins.

Greek

Nearly 75 percent of all medical terms have Greek origins because the Ancient Greeks observed, described, and documented anatomy and pathology. In addition, the Greek language lends itself to easily connecting words, which is very useful for medical terms. That is how we can build a term as long and complex as "esophagogastroduodenoscopy" (more about this word, commonly abbreviated to "EGD," in a later chapter). It would be much harder to do this in other languages that don't use the same connecting vowels. If you see a long word with multiple root words back-to-back, it is likely Greek.

Latin

As the Romans took over Europe, Latin became the dominant language. As a result, many Greek medical terms were adapted into Latin. In fact, Latin was the preferred language of the sciences throughout the Western world until the 1800s. Since Latin has unique linguistic conventions, many of the terms were slightly modified. For instance, the letter "k" does not exist in Latin as it does in Greek, so words like "kranion" (Greek for "skull") became "cranium" when converted to Latin. Also, Greek commonly uses "ai" "and "oi," but Latin uses "ae" and "oe," so a Greek word like "diaita" became "diaeta" and eventually "diet." Similarly, the Greek suffixes "os" and "on" became "us" and "um," so the Greek "bacterion" became "bacterium."

Examples

On the rare occasion, you will run into medical synonyms, or multiple terms that mean the same thing. The study of the kidneys is called both "nephrology" (Greek) and "renal" (Latin). The belly button can be called both "omphalo-" (Greek) and "umbilicus" (Latin). To describe the womb, both "hyster-" (Greek) and "uter-" (Latin) are used. There are only a handful of examples in which terms exist in both languages, and I will be sure to point those out. Fortunately, you don't need to learn Greek and Latin for every medical term.

HOW TO PLURALIZE TERMS

In English, we typically indicate plurality by putting an "s" at the end of a word. For example, more than one knee is "knees." Because medical terms originated from Greek and Latin, changing a word from singular to plural is a little more complicated. I recommend making these pluralization rules into flash cards. As you encounter medical terms in the next chapters, pay attention to whether they are in the singular or plural form and guess what the word would be in the opposite form. There are exceptions, but these rules apply nearly 99 percent of the time.

IF THE SINGULAR ENDS IN	EXAMPLE	TO MAKE IT PLURAL	EXAMPLE
a	patella (knee bone)	add an **e**	patellae
ax	thorax (chest)	remove the **ax** and add **ces**	thoraces
ex	cortex	remove **ex** and add **ces**	cortices
is	diagnosis	remove the **is** and add **es**	diagnoses
itis	vasculitis (inflammation of the arteries)	remove the s and add **des**	vasculitides
ix	appendix	remove the **ix** and add **ces**	appendices

(continued)

(continued from previous page)

IF THE SINGULAR ENDS IN	EXAMPLE	TO MAKE IT PLURAL	EXAMPLE
ma	stoma (opening)	add **ta** to make it plural	stomata
on	ganglion (a cluster of nerve cells)	remove **on** and add **ia**	ganglia
um	atrium (heart chamber)	remove **um** and add **ia**	atria
us	thrombus (blood clot)	remove **us** and add **i**	thrombi
us	viscus (internal organ)	remove **us** and add **era**	viscera
x	phalanx (the bone of a toe or finger)	remove the **x** and add **ges**	phalanges
y	biopsy	remove the **y** and add **ies**	biopsies

GETTING STARTED

You might already feel overwhelmed, and that is perfectly normal at this point. Remember that you are learning a new language, and immersing yourself in a language accelerates your ability to learn it. By developing a strong foundation of the origins of medical terms (the building blocks of prefixes, root words, and suffixes) and understanding how to change between singular and plural, you'll be well on your way to fluency.

It may take you a couple of weeks to memorize each of the sections in this book, but I promise that the process will become second nature much sooner than you realize. I also recommend practicing good sleep hygiene as you pursue this learning experience. You will find that when you wake up from a good night's sleep or even a power nap, you remember quite a bit more than when you fell asleep. This is because deep sleep allows the brain to make connections between neurons, also known as neural networks ("neuro" being a root word referring to nerves and the nervous system).

KEY TAKEAWAYS

This chapter's goal was to lay the foundation for your understanding of medical terminology. I recommend that you become confident in the terms and rules from this chapter before moving on to chapter 2, as each chapter builds on the information from previous chapters. I also suggest creating flash cards for both the rules of pronunciation and how to convert terms from singular to plural. Here are four key takeaways from this chapter:

- All medical terms can be broken into components: prefix, root, and suffix. When you understand the meaning of these components, you will have the ability to master larger, more complex words.

- There are certain pronunciation rules that apply to medical terminology; with practice, you will be able to articulate them correctly.

- Medical terms have their origins in Ancient Greek and Latin. Even though these terms can seem complicated, they are actually very basic once you understand the translations.

- There are rules that define how Greek and Latin words are converted from singular to plural. Use flash cards to commit this key information to memory.

QUIZ

1. In the term "echocardiogram," which is the root word?

   a. echo

   b. cardio

   c. gram

2. In the term "transesophageal," which is the suffix?

   a. trans

   b. esophag

   c. eal

3. How do you pronounce "cholecystitis"?

   a. CHOO-lee-kiss-EYE-tis

   b. KOLL-ee-sist-EYE-tis

   c. choo-luh-sys-EAT-iss

4. What is the origin of the word "ophthalmology"?

   a. Greek

   b. Latin

5. What is the origin of the word "cervix"?

   a. Greek

   b. Latin

6. What is the plural form of "pneumothorax"?

   a. pneumothoraxes

   b. pneumothoraces

   c. pneumothori

   d. pneumothora

7. What is the singular form of "viscera"?

   a. visceri

   b. viscero

   c. viscerum

   d. viscer

8. What is the singular form of "vasculitides"?

   a. vascula

   b. vasculite

   c. vasculitis

   d. vasculum

ANSWERS

1. b 2. c 3. b 4. a 5. b 6. b 7. c 8. c

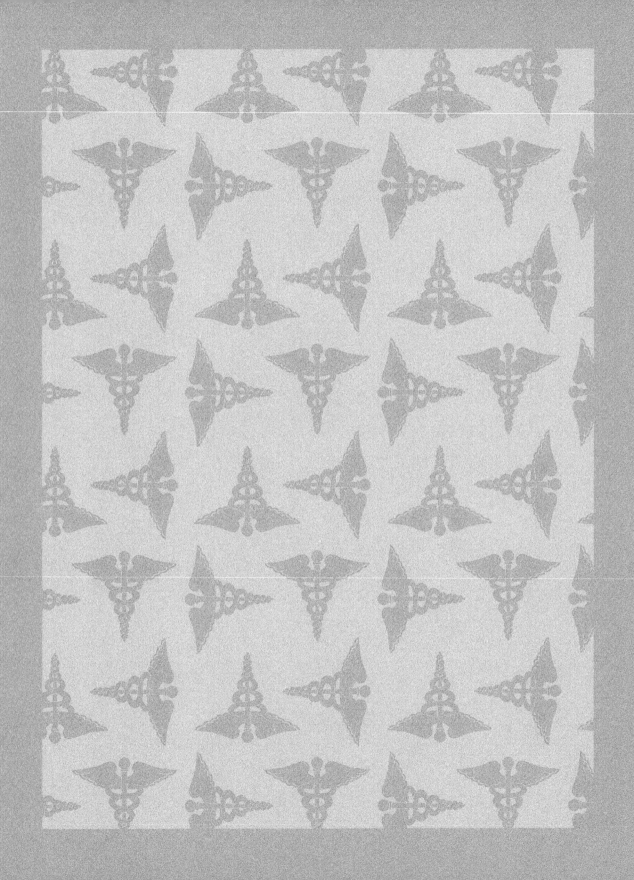

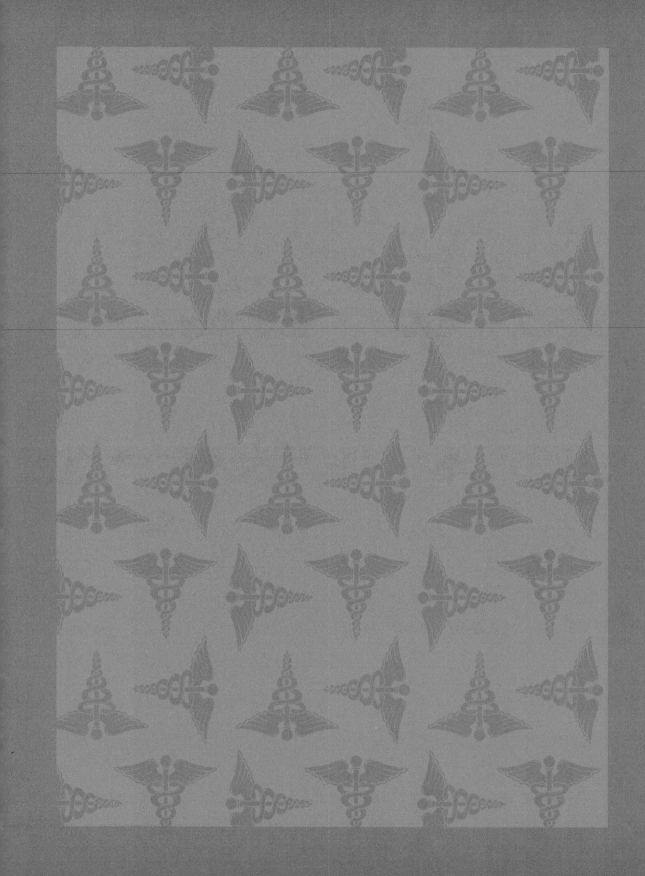

CHAPTER 2

HOW THE BODY IS ORGANIZED

Now we are ready to start learning medical terminology. In my training, I have found it best to start broad and then zoom in on the finer details. Before learning the actual organs and organ systems, we must first examine how the body can be viewed and divided. We'll begin by learning the planes and positions. These concepts are especially relevant for radiologists, who use images in these planes for diagnoses.

We will then explore the major body regions and cavities, such as the chest, abdomen, and pelvis. The abdomen will then be further divided because, in clinical medicine, we often think of abdominal pathology in regard to the affected "quadrant" or "subregion" to better understand the source of the ailment. By the end of this chapter, you will understand how the body is oriented and positioned, which will give you the lay of the land as we take a closer look in the chapters to come.

PLANES AND POSITIONS

The human body can be viewed and examined in a variety of ways. When learning anatomy, reading radiology images, or performing an autopsy, the body can be virtually (or literally) "sliced" in various planes. There are medical terms that describe all of these planes and positions.

In case it has been a while since your study of geometry, a plane is a flat surface. Anatomic planes are the various ways the body can be viewed in cross-section. It may sound a little gruesome, but to conceptualize anatomical planes, you can imagine that you have a very large, sharp knife that allows you to make a clean cut through the body. Each plane slices the body in a different direction or angle. Computed Tomography (CT) scanning and Magnetic Resonance Imaging (MRI), for example, use computer processing to create images in various anatomical planes. This allows radiologists to examine the body, slice by slice, to better view internal structures and make diagnoses.

ANATOMICAL PLANES

There are three main planes in which to view the body. Think of each plane as a sheet of glass that slices through the body. With half of the body removed, you could look directly at the internal structures from a specific vantage point. Classically, these planes pass through the exact midline of the body. However, in radiographic imagery, the location of the plane, or the "cut," can be shifted or tilted up or down, front to back, and left to right.

ANATOMICAL PLANES	
NAME	DESCRIPTION
Axial plane	Also known as the horizontal or transverse plane, the axial plane divides the body into superior (upper) and inferior (lower) parts. This is a very common plane in which to view CT scans, particularly of the head, chest, abdomen, and pelvis.

ANATOMICAL PLANES	
NAME	DESCRIPTION
Coronal plane	Otherwise known as the frontal plane, the coronal plane is the vertical plane that separates the human body into anterior (front) and posterior (back) portions. Imagine the slice begins where a crown ("corona") would sit on your head.
Sagittal plane	The sagittal, or median, plane is the vertical plane that divides the body into left and right halves. This is a very useful plane for radiologists to review CT scans and MRIs, especially if they are investigating the vertebrae, spinal cord, and nerve roots.

BODY POSITIONS

In clinical medicine, there are various ways in which a patient can be positioned. This becomes very relevant for physical examinations and surgical procedures. Having specific medical terminology for body positions is helpful for fast and reliable communication. It is much easier to ask the nurse to position the patient in "left lateral decubitus" position than it is to say, "Can you put the patient on their side with their legs straight and left arm supporting their head?"

BODY POSITIONS	
NAME	DESCRIPTION
Anatomic position	Considered the "standard position" (Imagine a person standing in front of you, head facing forward, feet planted on the floor with palms facing your direction.)
Supine or dorsal recumbent	Lying face up, on the back
Fowler	Lying supine with the head of the bed elevated at roughly 45 to 60 degrees to create a semi-seated position
Lateral recumbent or lateral decubitus	Lying on the side (either left or right), with knees slightly bent and lower arm supporting the head

(continued)

(continued from previous page)

BODY POSITIONS	
NAME	DESCRIPTION
Lithotomy	A specific position for pelvic exams and procedures in which the patient is positioned supine with bent knees and thighs drawn toward the abdomen
Prone	Lying face down, on the belly
Reverse Trendelenburg	Lying supine with legs lowered slightly below head level
Trendelenburg	Lying supine with legs raised slightly higher than head level

BODY DIRECTIONS

When describing anatomy, it is essential to be able to specify location and direction. Imagine being in a new city, trying to navigate with a map. You rely on using directional terms such as "north," "south," "east," "west," "next to," and "across from." The same holds true in medicine, in which specific terms describe direction, orientation, and relative position.

Note: You'll see the term "axial skeleton" in this chart; this term refers to bones of the head, spine, and rib cage. The "appendicular skeleton" consists of the bones of the upper and lower limbs, pelvis, and shoulders.

BODY DIRECTIONS	
NAME	DESCRIPTION
Anterior (an-TEER-ee-err)	Toward the front of the body
Caudal (CAW-dle)	Toward the tail (or tailbone); often used interchangeably with "inferior" but does not apply if referring to a structure below the tailbone
Cranial (KRAY-nee-uhl)	Toward the head; often used interchangeably with "superior"
Deep (DEEP)	Farther away from the surface or closer to the absolute center of the body
Distal (DISS-tull)	Farther away from the axial skeleton; often referring to structures of the limbs

BODY DIRECTIONS	
NAME	DESCRIPTION
Dorsal (DOOR-sull)	The backside; also refers to the back of the hand and the top of the foot (This can be remembered by visualizing any part of the body that would directly get wet during a rainstorm if you walked on all fours.)
External (ex-TER-nal)	Outside or outer
Inferior (in-FEAR-ee-or)	Down, or below; often used interchangeably with "caudal"
Internal (in-TER-null)	Inside or inner
Lateral (LAT-err-all)	Away from the midline (from the sagittal plane)
Medial (ME-dee-all)	Toward the midline (from the sagittal plane)
Palmar (PALM-arr)	The palm side of the hand
Plantar (PLAN-tar)	The sole of the foot (the side planted into the ground when standing)
Posterior (post-EAR-ee-or)	Toward the backside of the body (from the coronal plane)
Proximal (PROX-ih-mull)	Closer to the axial skeleton; often refers to structures of the limbs
Superficial (soup-err-FISH-ull)	Closer to the surface
Superior (soup-EAR-ee-or)	Up, above, or toward the head; also called "cranial"

BODY REGIONS AND CAVITIES

The human body has two large cavities, the thorax and abdomen. Technically, there is also a cranial cavity (inside the skull) and a pelvic cavity, but we will focus on the two largest. The word "cavity" comes from the latin "cavus," which means "hollow" and is also the origin of the word "cave." The thorax and abdomen are two relatively large spaces that are filled with vital organs. The structure separating the thorax from the abdomen is the diaphragm, the large, flat muscle that allows us to take a breath in. Above the diaphragm is the thorax, and below is the abdomen.

The abdomen can be subdivided into quadrants and regions. As the name suggests, there are four *quad*rants, and less obvious, there are nine abdominal regions. Note that there are no actual physical barriers that create these separations. These subdivisions help primarily with diagnosis because each organ, when afflicted, tends to express pain in a particular quadrant or region. Also, keep in mind that quadrants and regions are two different ways to divide the same area. Clinicians choose which convention works best for them in each situation. I use both depending on the clinical scenario.

In addition to body regions, it is important to know the five regions of the spine, or backbone (more detail will be explained later on). They are listed here, starting cranially (toward the head) and moving caudally (toward the tail):

Cervical, from Latin "cervix," meaning "neck." There are **7** cervical vertebrae, denoted C1-C7. C1 is also known as the "atlas" and C2 as the "axis." These two vertebrae are critical support structures for the human skull.

Thoracic, from Greek "thōrakikós," meaning "chest." There are **12** thoracic vertebrae, denoted T1-T12.

Lumbar, from Latin "lumbus," meaning "loin." There are **5** lumbar vertebrae (L1-L5).

Sacral, from Latin "sacralis," meaning "sacred." Clinically, the sacral region has incredibly complex and important anatomy. There are **5** sacral vertebrae, fused into one solid heart-shaped bone.

Coccyx, from Greek "kokkux," meaning "cuckoo" because the bone resembles the shape of the cuckoo bird's beak. The coccyx is often called the "tailbone" but is actually **3–5** tiny vertebrae fused together.

ANTERIOR BODY PARTS

There are many terms for regions of the body; often they relate to particular organs or body parts. Here is a list of the regions that can be viewed from the anterior, or front side of the body. I've sorted them by the overarching body region for easier understanding and memorization.

ANTERIOR BODY REGIONS		
NAME AND PRONUNCIATION	COMMON NAME	REGION
Abdomen (ab-DOH-men)	Belly	Abdomen/Pelvis
Inguinal (in-GWIN-uhl)	Groin	Abdomen/Pelvis
Pubic (PYOO-bick)	Pubic	Abdomen/Pelvis
Umbilical (um-BILL-ick-uhl)	Belly button	Abdomen/Pelvis
Cephalic (SEFF-a-lick)	Head	Head and neck
Cervical (SIR-vic-uhl)	Neck	Head and neck
Cranial (CRAY-nee-uhl)	Skull	Head and neck
Facial (FAY-shull)	Face	Head and neck
Frontal (FRONT-uhl)	Forehead	Head and neck
Nasal (NAZE-uhl)	Nose	Head and neck
Oral (OR-uhl)	Mouth	Head and neck
Orbital (or-BIT-uhl), **Ocular** (OCK-you-lar)	Eyes	Head and neck
Temporal (temp-OR-uhl)	Side of head	Head and neck
Crural (CREW-rall)	Leg	Lower extremities
Femoral (FEM-or-uhl)	Thigh	Lower extremities
Hallus (HALL-iss)	Big toe	Lower extremities
Patellar (pat-ELL-err)	Kneecap	Lower extremities
Pedal (PEE-dull)	Foot	Lower extremities

(continued)

(continued from previous page)

ANTERIOR BODY REGIONS		
NAME AND PRONUNCIATION	COMMON NAME	REGION
Tarsal (TAR-suhl)	Ankle	Lower extremities
Axillary (AX-ih-lair-ee)	Armpit	Thorax
Costal (COST-uhl)	Ribs	Thorax
Deltoid (DELL-toid)	Shoulder	Thorax
Mammary (MAM-ma-ree)	Breast	Thorax
Pectoral (PECK-tor-uhl)	Chest	Thorax
Sternal (STER-nuhl)	Breastbone	Thorax
Subxiphoid (sub-ZYE-foid)	Below breastbone	Thorax
Thoracic (thor-A-sic)	Chest	Thorax
Antebrachial (ANT-ee-BRAKE-ee-uhl)	Forearm	Upper extremities
Antecubital (ANT-ee-CUBE-it-uhl)	Front of elbow	Upper extremities
Brachial (BRAKE-ee-uhl)	Arm	Upper extremities
Carpal (KARP-uhl)	Wrist	Upper extremities
Hypothenar (hi-poh-THEE-nar)	Little finger	Upper extremities
Palmar (PALM-arr)	Palm	Upper extremities
Phalangeal (FAY-lan-GEE-uhl)	Digits	Upper extremities
Thenar (THEE-nar)	Thumb	Upper extremities

POSTERIOR BODY PARTS

Imagine now that you are viewing the body from the posterior (or back) side. The following table outlines all of the posterior anatomic subregions. For most of these, if you remove the ending "al," these terms can be used as root words.

POSTERIOR BODY REGIONS		
NAME AND PRONUNCIATION	COMMON NAME	REGION
Occipital (ock-SIP-ih-tall)	Posterior head	Head and neck
Parietal (puh-RYE-ih-tall)	Mid-posterior/lateral head	Head and neck
Calcaneal (cal-CANE-ee-all)	Heel	Lower extremities
Plantar (PLANT-arr)	Sole of foot	Lower extremities
Popliteal (pop-lit-EE-uhl)	Back of knee	Lower extremities
Sural (SIR-uhl)	Calf region	Lower extremities
Tarsal (TAR-sull)	Ankle	Lower extremities
Coccygeal (COX-eh-GEE-uhl)	Tailbone	Pelvis
Gluteal (gloot-EE-uhl)	Buttocks	Pelvis
Perineal (pair-ih-NEE-uhl)	Between genitals and anus	Pelvis
Sacral (SAKE-rall)	Between hips	Pelvis
Dorsal (DORR-sall)	Back, including back of hand	Thorax
Iliac (ILL-ee-ack)	Hip/waist	Thorax
Lumbar (LUM-bar)	Low back	Thorax
Vertebral (ver-TEE-brall)	Spinal column	Thorax
Cutibal (CUBE-it-uhl)	Elbow	Upper extremities
Scapular (SCAP-you-lar)	Shoulder blade	Upper extremities

QUADRANTS OF THE ABDOMEN

As you'll see, certain organs or portions of organs are located in specific quadrants. During a physical exam, a health-care provider will inspect, auscultate (or listen), percuss (tap on), and palpate (press) lightly and deeply in each of these quadrants. Eliciting pain or discomfort in a particular quadrant can help a clinician make a diagnosis. In clinical practice, we often use abbreviations to quickly refer to the abdominal quadrants. For instance, a clinician may ask, "Did the patient have any RUQ tenderness?" Another may reply, "No, but they were guarding their LLQ." The abbreviations are in parentheses below.

QUADRANTS OF THE ABDOMEN	
NAME	ASSOCIATED ORGANS
Right upper quadrant (RUQ)	Gallbladder, right lobe of the liver, biliary ducts, head of pancreas, right kidney, right adrenal gland, "hepatic flexure" of colon
Left upper quadrant (LUQ)	Stomach, left lobe of the liver, spleen, body of pancreas, left kidney, left adrenal gland, "splenic flexure" of colon
Right lower quadrant (RLQ)	Ileum (distal small intestine), ascending colon and cecum, appendix, right ureter, right ovary/fallopian tube
Left lower quadrant (LLQ)	Descending and sigmoid colon, left ureter, left ovary/fallopian tube

NINE REGIONS OF THE ABDOMINAL-PELVIC AREA

While most clinicians, including myself, primarily use the abdominal quadrants, some, mostly general surgeons, prefer referencing the nine abdominal-pelvic regions. The quadrants and regions cover roughly the same area, except that the nine regions also include the pelvis. Dividing the abdomen into nine regions allows for more precise analysis and diagnosis. Hint: If you are working on a surgical unit, use the nine regions.

You'll notice the word "hypochondriac" included here. That term is commonly used to describe someone who insists they are always sick. The origin of the term is interesting; it means "melancholy without real cause." Ancient doctors believed that the organs in the "hypochondriac" region were responsible for "melancholy," or "black bile" ("melano" + "chole"). Don't be deceived by the name; there are many illnesses that originate in this region.

REGIONS OF THE ABDOMINAL-PELVIC AREA		
REGION	LOCATION	ASSOCIATED ORGANS
Right hypochondriac region	Upper right part of abdomen, specifically below the lower rib cage	Gallbladder, right lobe of liver, "hepatic flexure" of colon, small intestine, upper pole of right kidney, and right adrenal gland
Right lumbar region	Middle right part abdomen, at the same level as the lumbar spine	Ascending colon, small intestine, right kidney and proximal ureter
Right iliac region	Lower right part of abdomen, near the iliac crest	Appendix, ascending colon, cecum, small intestine (ileum)

(continued)

(continued from previous page)

REGIONS OF THE ABDOMINAL-PELVIC AREA		
REGION	LOCATION	ASSOCIATED ORGANS
Epigastric region	Above the stomach, below the breastbone	Liver, bile ducts, stomach, spleen, small intestine (duodenum), adrenal glands, pancreas
Umbilical region	Around the umbilicus (belly button or navel)	Small intestine (duodenum), transverse colon, abdominal aorta
Hypogastric region	Below the stomach, below the umbilicus	Bladder, sigmoid colon, small intestine, reproductive organs
Left hypochondriac region	Upper left part of abdomen, specifically below the lower rib cage	Liver (the leftmost tip), stomach, spleen, pancreas, left kidney, left adrenal gland, "splenic flexure" of colon, small intestine
Left lumbar region	Middle left part abdomen, at the same level as the lumbar spine	Descending colon, left kidney and proximal left ureter, small intestine
Left iliac region	Lower left part of abdomen, near the iliac crest	Descending colon, sigmoid colon, small intestine

FIVE REGIONS OF THE SPINE

The spinal column is also known as the "vertebral column" or "backbone." It is made of 33 vertebrae, 24 of which are distinct (separate) bones in the cervical, thoracic, and lumbar spine. The sacrum has five vertebrae that fuse together soon after birth. The coccyx most commonly is made of four fused vertebrae but can have between three and five.

REGIONS OF THE SPINE			
REGION	ABBREVIATION	ROOT WORD, MEANING	LOCATION
Cervical region	C-spine	Cervic, neck	Neck area, composed of seven vertebrae labeled C1 to C7
Thoracic region	T-spine	Thora, chest	Upper back, composed of twelve vertebrae labeled T1 to T12
Lumbar region	L-spine	Lumb, loin	Lower back, composed of five vertebrae labeled L1 to L5
Sacral region	S	Os sacrum, "holy bone"	Between the hips, five fused vertebrae labeled S1-S5
Coccygeal region	N/A	Kokkux, cuckoo (resembles the beak of a cuckoo bird)	The tailbone is actually three to five fused vertebrae at the end of the spinal column.

VENTRAL CAVITY SUBDIVISIONS

The ventral cavity is filled with many internal organs. It is subdivided into the chest, abdomen, and pelvis. The diaphragm muscle physically separates the thorax from the abdomen. The abdomen and pelvis are not physically divided, but the space enclosed by the pelvic bones is called the pelvic cavity.

VENTRAL CAVITY SUBDIVISIONS		
NAME	RELATED ROOT WORD	ORGANS
Thoracic cavity	Thorac/o	Trachea, lungs, heart, aorta, and esophagus
Abdominal cavity	Abdomin/o	Stomach, small intestine, large intestine, liver, gallbladder, biliary ducts, pancreas, spleen, kidneys, adrenal glands, appendix, abdominal aorta, inferior vena cava
Pelvic cavity	Pelvic/o	Bladder, rectum, reproductive organs

DORSAL CAVITY SUBDIVISIONS

Compared to the ventral cavities, which contain many organs, the dorsal cavities are much smaller and only contain elements of the central nervous system (the brain and spinal cord). That being said, these cavities are incredibly important. An injury to the brain or spinal cord can be catastrophic.

DORSAL CAVITY SUBDIVISIONS		
NAME	RELATED ROOT WORD	ORGANS
Cranial cavity	Crani/o = Relating to the skull and contents within	The brain and meninges
Spinal cavity (or canal)	Spinal = Relating to the spinal cord and surrounding structures	The spinal cord, meninges, and nerve roots

KEY TAKEAWAYS

You made it to the end of chapter 2. The goal of this chapter was to learn how the body is organized. We outlined the various planes from which the body can be visualized for the study of anatomy or in clinical practice by a radiologist. We then discussed the major cavities of the chest, abdomen, and pelvis. We learned how to divide the abdomen into four quadrants or nine regions to better understand the anatomy. We explored all five regions of the spinal column, then finished by discussing the ventral (or anterior) and dorsal (or posterior) body cavities. In other words, you've mapped out the entire human body.

Now that you've learned your way around, you are ready for some more in-depth exploration of the body's organ systems and the terms that describe them. But first, here are four key takeaways from this chapter:

- The body can be viewed in three basic, often theoretical, planes: axial, coronal, and sagittal.

- The body can be divided into anterior and posterior regions and subregions.

- There are three ventral cavities—the chest, abdomen, and pelvis—and two dorsal cavities—the cranium (skull) and spinal canal.

- The abdomen can be divided into four quadrants or nine regions. If you are working on a surgical unit, refer to the nine regions, as it's more precise.

QUIZ

1. Which plane divides the body into front and back sections?

   a. axial/transverse

   b. coronal

   c. sagittal/midsagittal

2. Which plane divides the body into superior and inferior sections?

   a. axial/transverse

   b. coronal

   c. sagittal/midsagittal

3. Which body position refers to a patient lying on their back with their feet elevated slightly above their head?

   a. trendelenburg

   b. prone

   c. fowler

4. The nose is _____ to the eyes.

   a. lateral

   b. medial

   c. superior

5. The hand is ___ to the elbow.

   a. proximal

   b. superior

   c. distal

6. What is the medical term for the head region?

   a. cervical

   b. cranial

   c. caudal

7. What is the medical term for the foot region?

   a. plantar

   b. pedal

   c. crural

8. What is the medical term for the posterior knee region?

   a. plantar

   b. femoral

   c. popliteal

9. The appendix is most commonly located in which abdominal quadrant?

   a. RUQ

   b. LLQ

   c. RLQ

10. Which abdominal region refers to "below the left ribcage?"

    a. epigastric

    b. left lumbar

    c. left hypochondriac

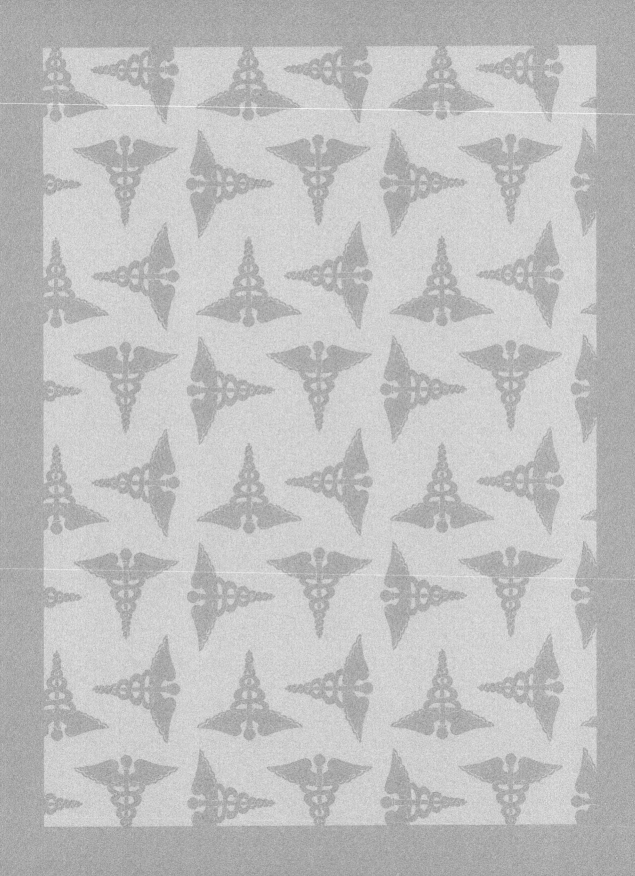

pan stasis physis

ipsi septo intus

tort ileo hepat

intra chondro pe

neuro cyte vas

deno ular c

chole itis sarco t

rectomy cephalo

dema esis trophy

sarcoma osis

pseudo xeno le

oxy thorac hydr

andr cili ren cephal

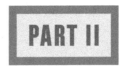

PART II

MEDICAL TERMS BY ROOT, PREFIX, AND SUFFIX

In chapter 1, I explained the importance of learning prefixes, root words, and suffixes. Learning these word components will exponentially increase your medical vocabulary. For example, if you learn three prefixes, three root words, and three suffixes, you've gained nine new terms. However, there are also twenty-seven theoretical combinations of those terms. And that doesn't include combining root words with each other (as in cardiopulmonary or hepatorenal). Of course, not all possible combinations will yield words that are commonly used in medicine, but many will. By focusing on mastering these components rather than memorizing long lists of words, you'll develop a vocabulary that grows quickly and keeps expanding. You'll see terms you have never encountered before and be able to understand their meaning. By the time you finish this book, you'll be able to create and understand thousands of medical terms.

This is going to take some work. All worthwhile things in life do. But with focused effort, wellness breaks, healthy food, and restful sleep, anyone can do it. Get out those flash cards or pull out your smartphone and open your favorite study app, because it's time to start learning.

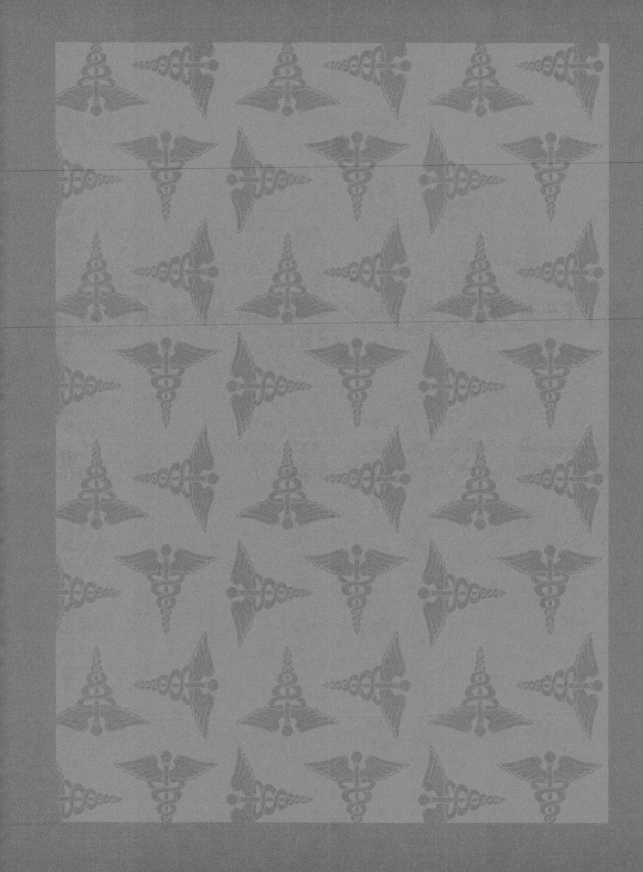

CHAPTER 3

ROOT WORDS OF THE BODY'S SYSTEMS

We are about to dive into the root words that describe the body's major organ systems, such as the cardiovascular system (heart and blood vessels) and the respiratory system (lungs and airways). Grouping the terms by each organ system will enhance your understanding and retention, since each organ system has terminology relating to its unique structure and function. Physicians and scientists tend to specialize in a particular system, and many medical schools teach curricula in an organ-system based manner to facilitate learning. I recommend you spend time learning the vocabulary of each organ system before moving on to the next one.

I mentioned a key rule earlier that's worth repeating here: many medical terms, particularly those of Greek origin, connect subunits with the letter "o." This particularly holds true if the second part of a series begins with a consonant. The words "cardiopulmonary" or "bronchopleural" are great examples of this. So, you'll see each term listed with and without the trailing "o." Take note of where the "o" connectors are, and are not, used throughout this chapter.

It is also important to understand that the root word does not always occur in the middle of a term. Sometimes it's at the beginning or end. Think of the root as the core of the word, what gives it significance and context, regardless of where it's positioned. Cardiology, for instance, is the study of the heart, and "cardio" is the root despite it being the first portion of the term. This will make more sense as we go along, but just keep in mind, these terms are flexible in their organization.

ROOT WORDS OF THE CARDIOVASCULAR SYSTEM

The cardiovascular (CAR-dee-oh-VAS-cue-lar) system is made of the heart (cardio) and blood vessels (vascular). Since cardiovascular disease is so widespread, it's likely many of these terms are already familiar to you. Let's look at some of the most important root words in this organ system.

THE CARDIOVASCULAR SYSTEM		
ROOT WORD	MEANING	EXAMPLE
Angi/o (ANN-gee-oh)	Blood vessel (more commonly referring to arteries than veins)	Angiogram, a procedure that examines arteries
Aort/o (AY-ort)	Relating to the aorta, the largest artery in the body	Aortitis, inflammation in the walls of the aorta
Arteri/o (ar-TEER-ee)	Relating to arteries	Arteriosclerosis, thickening and hardening of arterial walls
Ather/o (ATH-err)	Yellow, fatty substance that builds up in arteries	Atherectomy, a procedure to remove plaque from an artery
Atri/o (AY-tree)	Relating to the heart's atria (the two superior heart chambers; single = atrium)	Atriocaval, the location where the heart's right atrium meets the vena cavae (the body's largest veins)

THE CARDIOVASCULAR SYSTEM		
ROOT WORD	MEANING	EXAMPLE
Cardi/o (CAR-dee)	Relating to the heart	Cardiomyopathy, a condition in which the heart muscle is weakened
Diastol/e (dye-AS-toe-lee)	When the heart muscle is relaxed	Diastolic pressure, the blood pressure when the heart is relaxed
Phleb/o* (FLEB)	Relating to veins	Phlebotomy, removing blood from a vein, often called "a blood draw"
Systol/e (SIS-toe-lee)	When the heart muscle is contracting	Systolic pressure, the blood pressure when the heart is contracting
Tension (TEN-shunn)	Regarding blood pressure	Hypertension, high blood pressure; hypotension, low blood pressure
Valv/o (VALVE), **valvul/o** (VAL-view-lo)	Relating to the heart valves	Valvuloplasty, a procedure to repair a damaged heart valve
Vas/o (VAZE), **Vascul/o** (VAS-cue-lo)	Relating to blood vessels (both veins and arteries)	Vasoconstriction, when a blood vessel becomes narrowed. Vasculopathy, diseases of the blood vessels
Ven/o* (VEEN)	Relating to veins	Venogram, a procedure that examines veins
Ventricul/o (ven-TRICK-you-lo)	Relating to the heart ventricles (the two inferior heart chambers)	Ventriculomegaly, when the muscular walls of the ventricles become thickened and enlarged

* "Phlebo" is derived from Greek and "Veno" is Latin. Both mean "vein."

ROOT WORDS OF THE RESPIRATORY SYSTEM

The study of the respiratory system is known as pulmonology (pulm-uh-NOLL-oh-gee). The following table contains root words for major respiratory anatomy and functions.

THE RESPIRATORY SYSTEM		
ROOT WORD	MEANING	EXAMPLE
Alveol/o (al-VEE-oll)	Relating to the alveoli, tiny air sacs found at the end of bronchioles	Alveolitis, inflammation of the alveoli
Atel/o- (AT-ell)	Incomplete development, growth, or expression	Atelectasis, incomplete expansion or collapse of a portion of the lungs
Bronch/i/io (BRON-kee)	Relating to the bronchi, the larger airways with cartilage-rimmed walls	Bronchoconstriction, narrowing of the large airways
Bronchiol/i (Bron-KEE-oll)	Relating to the bronchioles, the smaller airways that do not have cartilage-supported walls	Bronchiolitis, inflammation in the lung's small airways
Capn/o (CAP-no)	Relating to carbon dioxide	Hypercapnia, a dangerous condition when the blood has too much carbon dioxide
Laryng/o (La-RIN-go)	Relating to the larynx or "voice box"	Laryngectomy, a surgical procedure to remove the larynx
Nas/o* (NAY-zo)	Relating to the nose	Nasopharynx, where the nose meets the posterior pharynx
Ox/i (OX)	Relating to oxygen	Hypoxia, too little oxygen in the blood
Phren/o (FREN-oh)	Relating to the diaphragm, the major muscle of breathing	Phrenoplegia, Paralysis of the diaphragm

THE RESPIRATORY SYSTEM		
ROOT WORD	MEANING	EXAMPLE
Pleur/o (PLURR-oh)	Relating to the pleura, the lining inside the chest wall	Pleurodesis, a surgical procedure to attach the lung to the lining of the chest wall to prevent collapse
Pneum/o (NEW-mo)	Relating to the lung or to air	Pneumothorax, a condition in which the lung collapses
Rhin/o* (RHI-no)	Relating to the nose	Rhinoplasty, surgical augmentation of the nose
Sinus/o (SINE-us)	Relating to the sinuses, air-filled spaces in the skull	Rhinosinusitis, inflammation of the nose and sinuses
Spir/o (SPY-ro)	"Coil," or in the setting of breathing, the act of moving air	Inspiration, taking a breath in
Trache/o (TRAY-kee)	Relating to the trachea, the first and largest airway portion	Tracheostomy, a surgical procedure in which a hole is placed in the trachea to allow for breathing

* "Naso" is Latin and "Rhino" is Greek; both mean "nose." The word "rhinoceros" comes from the Greek words "rhin" (nose) and "keras" (horn). The latter is the origin of the word "keratin," the protein that makes skin, hair, and nails . . . and rhino horns.

ROOT WORDS OF THE DIGESTIVE SYSTEM

The digestive system is commonly called the "gastrointestinal system," but that is a little bit of a misnomer. "Gastro" means "stomach" and "intestine" means, well, "intestines." However, there's a lot more to the digestive system than these two organs. I included a mention of the spleen in this table, even though it is not technically a digestive organ, because it is integrally linked to the liver and it also helps consume and process blood products. Here is a list of the major digestive system root words.

THE DIGESTIVE SYSTEM		
ROOT WORD	MEANING	EXAMPLE
Append/o (app-END)	Appendix	Appendicitis, inflammation due to an infection within the appendix
Cec/o (SEEK)	Cecum, the first portion of the large intestine	Cecectomy, surgical removal of the cecum
Chol/e (KOLL-ee)	Bile and biliary structures (such as the gallbladder)	Cholelithiasis, gallstones
Col/o (KO-lo), **Colon/o** (ko-LON-oh)	Colon, also known as the large intestine	Colectomy, surgical removal of all or part of the colon
Dent/o- (DENT)	Teeth	Dentist, a doctor specializing in teeth
Duoden/o (doo-oh-DEEN or doo-ODD-en)	Duodenum, the first portion of the small intestine	Duodenitis, inflammation and irritation of the duodenum
Enter/o (en-TERR-oh)	Any part of the small intestine	Enterovirus, a viral pathogen that causes diarrhea primarily by irritating the small intestine
Esophag/o (eh-SAH-fah-go)	Esophagus	Esophagram, a study that investigates the structure of the esophagus
Gastr/o (GAS-tro)	Stomach	Gastrostomy, a surgical opening made in the stomach

THE DIGESTIVE SYSTEM		
ROOT WORD	MEANING	EXAMPLE
Hepat/o (heh-PAT-oh)	Liver	Hepatotoxin, a substance or condition that is directly toxic to the liver
Ile/o (ILL-ee-oh)	Ileum, the last portion of the small intestine	Ileocecal valve, a structure at the intersection of the ileum and the cecum (the beginning of the large intestine)
Jejun/o (juh-JOON-oh)	Jejunum, the second portion of the small intestine	Jejunostomy tube, a feeding tube inserted directly into the jejunum
Or/o (OR-oh)	Mouth	Oropharynx, the region where the oral cavity and pharynx meet
Pancreat/o (pan-cree-AT-oh)	Pancreas	Pancreatitis, inflammation of the pancreas
Pharyng/o (fare-IN-go)	Pharynx, the region posterior to the oral cavity	Pharyngitis, inflammation and infection of the pharynx
Proct/o (PROCK-to)	Anus or rectum	Proctoscopy, a procedure to visually examine the anus and rectum
Rect/o (RECK-to)	Rectum, the muscular organ that connects the colon to the anus	Rectosigmoid junction, the anatomical location where the rectum and sigmoid colon meet
Sial/o- (SYE-ale-oh)	Saliva, salivary glands	Sialorrhea, excessive saliva production
Sigmoid/o (sig-MOYD-oh)	The S-shaped, last portion of the large intestine	Sigmoidoscopy, diagnostic procedure to visually examine the sigmoid colon
Splen/o (SPLEN-oh)	Spleen	Splenomegaly, an enlarged spleen

ROOT WORDS OF THE ENDOCRINE SYSTEM

The endocrine system is a fascinating collection of organs and glands that regulate the body's hormones. The word endocrine is derived from the Greek words "endo," meaning "within," and "krine," which means "to secrete." Thus, the term signifies that endocrine glands primarily secrete hormones within the bloodstream. The major endocrine organs are the pituitary, thyroid, parathyroids, adrenals, and gonads. We will discuss reproductive organ root words in later sections.

THE ENDOCRINE SYSTEM		
ROOT WORD	MEANING	EXAMPLE
Aden/o (AH-din-oh)	Gland, an organ that secretes a particular chemical substance	Adenocarcinoma, a malignant tumor made of glandular cells
Adren/o (uh-DREEN)	Adrenal gland	Adrenaline, a "fight or flight" hormone secreted by the adrenal glands, also known as epinephrine
Endocrin/o (EN-doh-krinn)	Relating to the glands that secrete hormones. Literally, "secreting inside" the bloodstream	Endocrinologist, a doctor who specializes in the body's hormones, hormone-producing organs, and their associated diseases
Gluc/o (GLOO-ko), **Glyc/o** (GLY-ko)	Glucose, blood sugar	Hyperglycemia, high blood sugar
Gonad/o (GO-nad)	Relating to the gonads, reproductive organs	Gonadotropin, a hormone secreted by the pituitary gland that stimulates ovaries and testes
Parathyr/o (pear-uh-THIGH-ro)	Pertaining to the four small parathyroid glands	Hyperparathyroidism, a condition in which one or all four parathyroid glands are overactive

THE ENDOCRINE SYSTEM		
ROOT WORD	MEANING	EXAMPLE
Pituitar/o (pit-OOH-ih-tare)	Pertaining to the pituitary gland	Hypopituitarism, a state in which the pituitary gland is producing insufficient amounts of hormones
Thyroid/o (THIGH-roid)	Thyroid gland	Hyperthyroidism, a state in which the thyroid is overactive

ROOT WORDS OF THE INTEGUMENTARY SYSTEM

The integumentary system refers to the body's largest organ system, the skin. Integument derives from the Latin "in," meaning "within," and "tegere," meaning "to cover." Thus, the integumentary system refers to the organs and tissues that cover the body. Doctors who specialize in the integumentary system are called dermatologists.

THE INTEGUMENTARY SYSTEM		
ROOT WORD	MEANING	EXAMPLE
Adip/o (AH-dip)	Body fat (adipose tissue) and fat cells	Adipocyte, a cell containing lipids
Cheil/o (KAI-lo)	Lips	Cheilosis, inflammation and irritation of the corners of the lips
Cutane/o (CUE-tane-ee)	Skin	Subcutaneous, below the epidermis and dermis
Derm/o (DERM), **Dermat/o** (dur-MAT-oh)	Skin	Intradermal, within the skin, often referring to a route of medication administration
Hidr/o (HI-dro)	Sweat glands	Hyperhidrosis, excessive sweating
Ichthy/o (ICK-thee)	"Fish-like," scaly	Ichthyosis, a condition of thickened, scale-like skin

(continued)

(continued from previous page)

THE INTEGUMENTARY SYSTEM		
ROOT WORD	MEANING	EXAMPLE
Kerat/o (ker-AT-oh)	Keratin, the protein that creates hair, skin, nails, and cornea.	Keratoconjunctivitis, inflammation and irritation of the front, exterior portion of the eye
Lip/o (LIP-oh)	Fat (adipose tissue) and fat cells	Liposuction, surgical removal of fat tissue
Onych/o (ON-ick-oh)	Nails	Onychomycosis, a fungal infection of the nails
Pil/o (PIE-lo)	Hair, or hair-like structures	Piloerection, when hair stands on end, also known as "goosebumps"
Seb/o (SEE-bo or SEB-oh)	Oil or sebum (an oily/waxy substance)	Sebaceous glands, oil-producing glands
Squamos/o- (SKWAY-mus)	Scaly or flaky; skin	Squamous cell, a thin, flat, skin cell
Ungu/o (UN-goo)	Nails	Subungual, underneath a finger or toenail
Trich/o (TRICK)	Hair	Trichotillomania, a psychological condition where a person has irresistible urges to pull out their own hair

ROOT WORDS OF THE MUSCULOSKELETAL SYSTEM

The musculoskeletal system comprises our muscles, bones, joints, and cartilage. These organs give our bodies support and structure and allow us to move. Many of these terms will be familiar to athletes and those who work in sports medicine or orthopedics.

THE MUSCULOSKELETAL SYSTEM		
ROOT WORD	MEANING	EXAMPLE
Ankyl/o (AN-kil-oh)	Crooked, bent, or fused	Ankylosis, abnormal stiffening of a joint
Arthr/o (ARTH-ro)	Relating to a joint or multiple joints	Arthrocentesis, a procedure to remove fluid from a joint space
Articul/o (are-TICK-you-lo)	Joint or movement	Articular cartilage, cartilage inside of joints
Burs/o (BURSE, like "purse")	Bursa, a fluid-filled sac that cushions joints	Bursitis, inflammation of the bursa
Carp/o (KARP)	Wrist area	Metacarpals, the five long bones of the hand
Chondr/o (CON-dro)	Cartilage	Chondrosarcoma, a malignant tumor of bone and cartilage cells
Cost/o (COST)	Ribs and the ribcage	Costochondritis, inflammation of the ribs and cartilage near the breastbone (sternum)
Femor/o (FEM-or)	Thigh	Femoroacetabular joint, also known as the hip joint, where the thigh bone (femur) meets the pelvic bone
Muscul/o (MUS-cue-lo)	Muscle	Musculoskeletal, the organ system consisting of muscles, connective tissues, and skeleton

(continued)

(continued from previous page)

THE MUSCULOSKELETAL SYSTEM		
ROOT WORD	MEANING	EXAMPLE
My/o (MY-oh)	Muscle	Myopathy, conditions in which muscles become weakened and deteriorate
Myel/o (MY-el-oh)*	Bone marrow	Myelofibrosis, a condition where bone marrow becomes scarred and no longer capable of producing essential blood cells
Osse/o (OSS-ee-oh), **Oste/o** (OSS-tee-oh)	Bone	Osteosarcoma, a malignant tumor of bones
Patell/o (Pa-TELL)	Knee bone	Patellofemoral Syndrome, a condition in which the cartilage under the kneecap is damaged
Pod/o (POD)	Foot	Podiatrist, a surgeon who specializes in the foot, ankle, and lower leg
Sarc/o (SARK-oh)	Flesh or muscle	Sarcopenia, loss of muscle mass or strength
Spondyl/o (SPON-dill-oh)	Vertebra (plural vertebrae, the bones of the spine)	Spondyloarthritis, an inflammatory condition affecting the spine
Stern/o (STERN-oh)	Sternum or breastbone	Sternoclavicular, the joint where the sternum (breastbone) meets the clavicle (collar bone)
Syn/o (SIN-oh)	Synovial joints, joints surrounded by a thick, flexible membrane that contains fluid	Synovitis, inflammation of synovial joints
Tal/o (TAIL-oh)	Ankle	Talocrural joint, the ankle joint

THE MUSCULOSKELETAL SYSTEM		
ROOT WORD	MEANING	EXAMPLE
Tars/o (TARS-oh)	Foot	Metatarsals, the five long bones of the foot
Ten/o (TEEN-oh)	Tendon	Tenosynovectomy, a surgical procedure to remove the tendon sheath
Tort/o (TORT-oh)	Twisted, spasm	Torticollis, a very painful muscle spasm of the neck
Vertebr/o (ver-TEE-bro)	Vertebra	Vertebroplasty, a procedure to stabilize a collapsed vertebra

* "Myel" comes from the Greek word "muelós" which means "marrow," or the soft, fleshy inside structures. The root "myel" refers to bone marrow and the spinal cord, both of which are soft, fatty, vascular tissues.

ROOT WORDS OF THE NERVOUS SYSTEM

The nervous system includes the brain, spinal cord, and peripheral nerves throughout the body. Not only does it control skeletal muscles that allow us to move, but it also controls our automatic bodily functions such as breathing and digestion.

THE NERVOUS SYSTEM		
ROOT WORD	MEANING	EXAMPLE
Aesthesi (as-THEE-zhuh)	Sensation	Anaesthesia, controlled reduction of sensation
Alge (al-GEE), **Algesia** (al-GEE-see-uh)	Pain	Analgesic, a drug or treatment to relieve pain
Cephal/o (CEFF-ah-lo)	Head or skull	Cephalohematoma, a bruise or collection of blood (heme) on the scalp
Cerebell/o (sare-eh-BELL)	Cerebellum, the area of the brain that controls coordination and balance	Cerebellopontine, the region of the brain where the cerebellum meets the brainstem (pons)
Cerebr/o (SIR-ee-br)	Relating to the cerebrum, the largest portion of the brain	Cerebritis, inflammation of the brain
Crani/o (CRAY-nee-oh)	Skull	Craniosynostosis, a birth anomaly in which a baby's skull plates fuse together prematurely
Encephal/o (en-CEFF-ah-lo)	Brain (or literally, "inside the skull")	Encephalopathy, when the brain is not functioning properly due to a disease or toxin
Gangli/o (GANG-lee-oh)	A cluster of nerve cell bodies	Ganglioma, a tumor or mass of nerve cells

THE NERVOUS SYSTEM		
ROOT WORD	MEANING	EXAMPLE
Mening/o (men-INN-go)	Relating to the meninges, membranes that surround the brain and spinal cord	Meningioma, a benign tumor of the meninges
Myel/o (MY-ell-oh)*	Spinal cord	Myelomalacia, a condition in which the spinal cord becomes softened or weakened
Neur/o (NURR-oh)	Nerves, nervous system	Neuropathy, nerve damage
Noci/o (NO-see)	Pain	Nociception, detection of painful stimuli
Psych/o (SYKE)	Mental, the mind	Psychiatry, the study of diagnosis, prevention, and treatment of mental disorders
Radicul/o (ra-DIK-you-lo)	Spinal nerve roots	Radiculopathy, injury to the spinal nerve roots
Somn/o (SOM-no)	Sleep	Hypersomnia, excessive sleeping
Spin/o (SPY-no)	Spine	Spinothalamic tract, nerve tracts that begin in the thalamus and extend the length of the spinal cord
Thym/o (THIGH-mo)	Emotion, or relating to the thymus (an organ)	Euthymic, pleasant and happy mood without disturbances

* "Myel/o" also refers to bone marrow, as mentioned in the previous chart.

ROOT WORDS OF THE SENSORY SYSTEM

As you know, we have five major senses: sight, smell, taste, hearing, and touch. Our bodies translate physical and chemical external stimuli into nerve impulses, and our brains use this information to create our sensory experiences. The following table provides root words for the organs, structures, and functions of the five major senses. Here are a few terms in this table that have both Greek and Latin versions:

Auri- (Latin) and oto- (Greek) for ear

Oculo- (Latin) and ophthalmo- (Greek) for eye

Lacrim- (Latin) and dacr- (Greek) for tear

Both versions of these terms are used commonly in medicine.

THE SENSORY SYSTEM		
ROOT WORD	MEANING	EXAMPLE
Audi/o (AW-dee-oh)	Sound or hearing	Auditory, relating to the sense of hearing
Auricul/o (or-ICK-you-lo)	Ear	Auriculoplasty, a cosmetic surgical procedure to adjust the shape of ears
Blephar/o (BLEH-far-oh)	Eyelid	Blepharospasm, abnormal contraction of the eyelid muscle causing eyelid twitching
Cochle/o (COKE-lee-oh)	The organ that transmits sound vibrations into nerve impulses	Cochlear implant, a surgical procedure to restore hearing by replacing the cochlea
Conjunctiv/o (con-junk-TIE-vo)	The mucus membrane that covers the front of the eye and lines the eyelids	Conjunctivitis, inflammation or infection of the conjunctiva, often called "pink eye"
Corne/o (cor-NEE-oh)	Cornea, the eye's clear protective outer layer	Corneal abrasion, a scratch of the cornea

THE SENSORY SYSTEM		
ROOT WORD	MEANING	EXAMPLE
Dacry/o (DACK-ro)	Tears and tear ducts	Dacryostenosis, a blocked tear duct causing dry eyes
Geus (GEESE, like cheese), **gust/o** (GUST-oh)	Sense of taste	Dysgeusia, altered sense of taste
Ir/o (EYE-ro), **irid/o** (ih-RID-oh)	Iris, the colored portion of the eye	Iridocyclitis, inflammation of the iris and surrounding structures seen in infections and autoimmune diseases
Labyrinth/o (LAB-ih-rinth-oh)	Bony structures of the inner ear that control hearing and equilibrium	Labrynthitis, inflammation of the inner ear
Lacrim/o (LACK-rim-oh)	Tear, tear duct	Lacrimorrhea, excessive tear production
Myring/o (mih-RING-oh)	Eardrum, also known as the tympanic membrane	Myringotomy, a surgical procedure to create a hole in the eardrum to allow fluid out
Ocul/o (OCK-you-lo)	Eye	Oculopathy, diseases of the eye
Olfact/o (oll-FACT-oh)	Sense of smell	Olfaction, the sense of smell
Ophthalm/o (OPP-thall-mo)	Eye	Ophthalmoscope, an instrument for inspecting the eye
Opt/o (OPT-oh)	Eye, vision	Optometrist, an eye doctor
Osmia (OZ-me-uh)	Sense of smell	Anosmia, loss of the sense of smell
Ot/o (OH-toe)	Ear	Otitis media, a middle ear infection
Phon/o (PHONE-oh)	Sound	Phonate, to produce or utter sounds

(continued)

(continued from previous page)

THE SENSORY SYSTEM		
ROOT WORD	MEANING	EXAMPLE
Phot/o (FOTE-oh)	Light	Photophobia, discomfort when looking at bright light
Tympan/o (tim-PAN-oh)	Eardrum (tympanic membrane)	Tympanostomy tubes, surgical tubes placed in the eardrum
Uve/o (YOU-vee-oh)	A group of structures in the front of the eye including the iris, ciliary body, and choroid plexus	Uveitis, inflammation of the uvea

ROOT WORDS OF THE URINARY SYSTEM

Medical doctors who specialize in diseases of the kidneys are known as nephrologists. Surgeons who specialize in the entire urinary system are known as urologists. Terms for the urinary or genitourinary (GU) system (the latter refers to the genitals and the organs responsible for urine production and elimination) can be a little confusing because some derive from Latin and others from Greek. As I mentioned earlier in this chapter, "renal" is Latin, and "nephro" is Greek, but both mean "kidneys."

THE URINARY SYSTEM		
ROOT WORD	MEANING	EXAMPLE
Azo/to (AY-zo)	Nitrogen-containing compound, often referring to blood urea nitrogen	Azotemia, elevated blood urea nitrogen levels
Cyst/o (SIST-oh)	Sac (bladder or gallbladder), or cyst	Cystoscopy, a procedure in which a small camera is used to look inside the bladder
Glomerul/o (glow-MER-you-lo)	Glomerulus (plural glomeruli), a complex microscopic structure in the kidneys	Glomerulonephritis, inflammation and damage to the glomeruli

THE URINARY SYSTEM		
ROOT WORD	MEANING	EXAMPLE
Lith/o (LITH-oh)	Stone	Nephrolithiasis, kidney stones
Nephr/o (NEFF-ro)	Kidney (Greek)	Nephrologist, a physician specializing in the kidneys
Pyel/o (PIE-el-oh)	Renal pelvis, the area of the kidney where urine is collected	Pyelonephritis, a serious bacterial infection of the renal pelvis
Ren/o (REEN-oh)	Kidney (Latin)	Renovascular hypertension, high blood pressure due to disease of the renal arteries
Ur/o (YURR-oh), **Urin/o** (YURR-in-oh)	Urine	Urosepsis, a severe urinary tract infection causing systemic illness Urinalysis, laboratory examination of a urine sample
Ureter/o (you-REE-ter-oh)	Ureter, the muscular tube that connects the kidneys to the bladder	Hydroureter, when the ureter becomes enlarged due to a blockage
Urethr/o (you-REETH-ro)	Urethra, the tube that leads from the bladder to the outside world	Urethroplasty, surgical repair of the urethra
Vesic/o (vess-ICK-oh)	Urinary bladder	Vesicoureteral reflux, inappropriate flow of urine from the bladder up the urethras

ROOT WORDS OF THE FEMALE REPRODUCTIVE SYSTEM

The following table includes commonly used root words relating to the female reproductive system. Note that in this and the following chart, the terms relate to biological sex and are not a commentary on gender. You will again notice some synonyms in both Greek and Latin.

THE FEMALE REPRODUCTIVE SYSTEM		
ROOT WORD	MEANING	EXAMPLE
Amni/o (am-NEE-oh)	Membranous fetal sac (amnionic sac)	Amniocentesis, removing fluid from the amniotic sac
Cervic/o (sir-VIC-oh)	Cervix, the "neck" of the uterus	Cervicitis, inflammation of the cervix
Colp/o (COLE-po)	Vagina (Greek)	Colposcopy, close examination of the vagina, cervix, and vulva for signs of disease
Endometri/o (en-doe-ME-tree-oh)	Endometrium, the inner lining of the uterus	Endometriosis, a painful condition in which endometrial tissue exists outside of the uterus
Episi/o (epp-EE-see-oh)	Vulva, the external female genitalia	Episiotomy, a tear in the vagina during childbirth
Galact/o (guh-LACT-oh)	Milk	Galactorrhea, milk flowing out of nipples other than during breast feeding
Gyn/o (GUY-no), **Gynec/o** (guy-NECK-oh)	Women, female	Gynecologist, a doctor who specializes in women's health, particularly of the reproductive organs
Hyster/o (HISS-ter-oh)	Uterus (Greek)	Hysterectomy, surgical removal of the uterus
Mamm/o (MAM-oh)	Breast (Latin)	Mammogram, a radiographic image of the breasts

THE FEMALE REPRODUCTIVE SYSTEM		
ROOT WORD	MEANING	EXAMPLE
Mast/o (MAST-oh)	Breast (Greek)	Mastitis, inflammation of the breast
Men/o (MEN-oh)	Month, monthly, menstrual cycle	Menorrhagia, heavy menstrual bleeding
Metr/o (MET-ro)	Uterus (Greek)	Metrorrhagia, bleeding between menstrual periods
Oophor/o (OO-for-oh)	Ovary, or "bearing eggs"	Oophorectomy, surgical removal of one or both ovaries
Ov/o (OH-vo)	Egg	Ovulation, the process of releasing an egg from the ovaries
Ovari/o (oh-VARE-ee-oh)	Ovaries	Ovaritis, inflammation of an ovary or ovaries
Salping/o (sal-PING-oh)	Fallopian tubes, the tubes that connect the ovaries to the uterus	Salpingectomy, a surgical procedure to remove the fallopian tubes
Uter/o (YOU-terr-oh)	Uterus (Latin)	Uterine fibroids, benign growths of the uterus
Vagin/o (VA-gin-oh)	Vagina	Vaginitis, inflammation of the vagina
Vulv/o (VULL-vo)	Vulva, the external female genitalia	Vulvodynia, chronic pain or discomfort around the opening of the vagina

ROOT WORDS OF THE MALE REPRODUCTIVE SYSTEM

The following are the major root words that refer to the male reproductive system. Note that the Greek and Latin roots for testicles are *orchi* and *test*, respectively. Interestingly, the Ancient Greeks thought testicles resembled orchid tubers and named them accordingly.

THE MALE REPRODUCTIVE SYSTEM		
ROOT WORD	MEANING	EXAMPLE
Andr/o (ANN-dro)	Male	Androgens, male sex hormones, such as testosterone
Balan/o (BALE-ann-oh)	Glans penis	Balanitis, inflammation and irritation of the glans penis
Epididym/o (ep-ih-DID-ee-mo)	Epididymis (plural epididymides), the duct that connects the testes to the vas deferens.	Epididymitis, infection within the epididymis
Orch/o (ORK-oh), **orchi/o** (ORK-ee-oh), **orchid/o** (ORK-id-oh)	Testes (Greek)	Orchiectomy, surgical removal of one or both testes
Phall/o (FAL-oh)	Phallus, penis	Phalloplasty, surgical construction or reconstruction of a penis
Prostat/o (pros-TAT-oh)	Prostate gland	Prostatectomy, surgical removal of the prostate gland
Scrot/o (SCROT-oh)	Scrotum	Scrotodynia, chronic pain of the scrotum
Test/o (TEST-oh), **testicul/o** (tes-TIC-you-lo)	Testis, testicle (Latin)	Testicular torsion, when a testicle twists around its blood supply

KEY TAKEAWAYS

That was a marathon of a chapter! By now, your flash cards must be well worn. On the bright side, you know a tremendous amount of frequently used medical terminology, including many root words from most major organ systems. In the next chapter, we will wrap up our study of root words with some critical terms that don't fall neatly into any organ systems yet are very important to have in your vocabulary. (For instance, we haven't covered hematology terms, which relate to the study of blood.) In the next section, we'll explore terms relating to both internal and external aspects of the body. Here are the key takeaways from this chapter:

* Many commonly used root words have both a Greek- and Latin-derived term. Latin roots tend to resemble English words more closely.

* Medical learning is best approached by grouping topics according to organ systems. This helps with memory retention.

* The cardiovascular, respiratory (or pulmonary), digestive, endocrine, integumentary, musculoskeletal, nervous, sensory, urinary, and reproductive systems all have specific root words relating to them.

QUIZ

1. What does the root word "phleb" refer to?
   a. phlegm
   b. veins
   c. valves

2. Fluid in the "space around the lungs" is called a _____ effusion.
   a. tracheal
   b. rhinal
   c. pleural

3. The hormone "cholecystokinin" causes which organ to contract?
   a. stomach
   b. spleen
   c. gallbladder

4. The term "hyperglycemia" means "high _____."
   a. blood sugar
   b. blood pressure
   c. glycerol

5. Which term refers to "goosebumps"?
   a. piloerection
   b. ichthyosis
   c. hyperhidrosis

6. Which term refers to muscle wasting?
   a. myoclonus
   b. sarcopenia
   c. chondritis

7. Inflammation of the membranes that surround the brain is called ___.
   a. meningitis
   b. cerebritis
   c. radiculitis

8. What would someone who has a "blepharoplasty" procedure might first complain of?

   a. droopy eyelids

   b. ugly nose

   c. big ears

9. The ureterovesicular junction is where the ureters enter the _____.

   a. kidneys

   b. intestine

   c. urinary bladder

10. The fallopian tubes allow eggs to pass from the ovaries to the _____, also known as the womb.

    a. uterus

    b. bladder

    c. vulva

11. "Orchitis" refers to an infection of the _____.

    a. kidneys

    b. penis

    c. testicles

ANSWERS

7. a   8. b   9. c   10. a   11. c

1. b   2. c   3. c   4. a   5. a   6. b

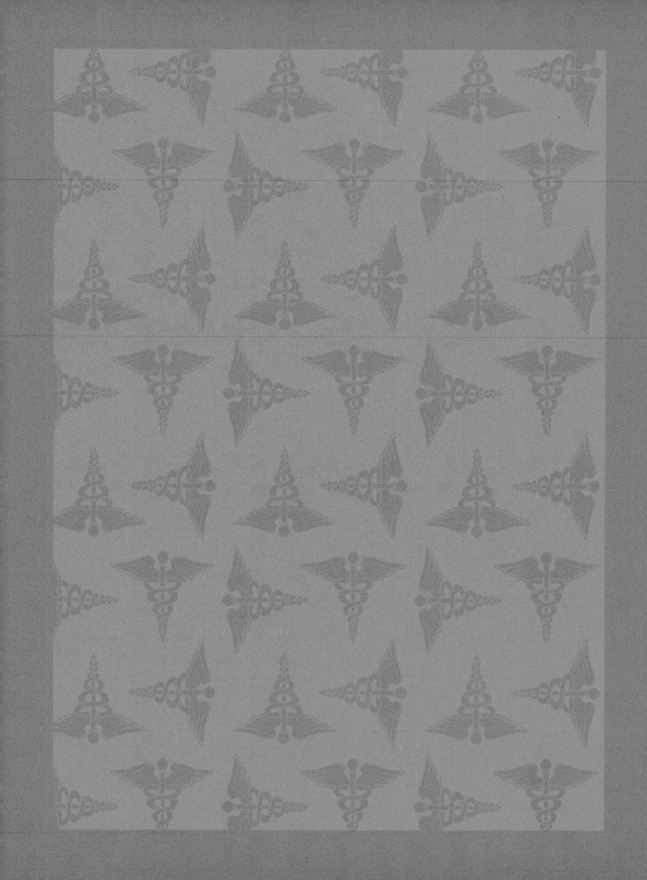

CHAPTER 4

ROOT WORDS FOR INTERNAL AND EXTERNAL BODY PARTS

There are many root words that don't fall neatly into organ systems but are very important to know. That makes for a bit of a potpourri chapter, but we'll organize these terms into external roots, internal roots, and directional words. External roots are words that apply to structures, regions, and body parts that are on the outside of the body, whereas internal roots relate to the inside of the body. This chapter includes words associated with direction and orientation that are very helpful in medical practice as well.

EXTERNAL ROOT WORDS

The following table contains terms relating to external body parts.

EXTERNAL ROOT WORDS		
ROOT WORD	MEANING	EXAMPLE
Acr/o (ACK-ro)	Tip, end, extremity	Acromegaly, a condition in which the body produces too much growth hormone, characterized by abnormally large hands and feet
Axill/o (ax-ILL-oh)	Armpit region	Axillary lymph nodes, lymph nodes in the armpit region
Blephar/o (BLEF-uh-ro)	Eyelid	Blepharoplasty, surgical modification of the eyelids
Brachi/o (BRAKE-ee-oh)	Arm	Brachial artery, the major artery of the arm
Bucc/o (BUCK-oh)	Cheek or mouth	Buccal mucosa, the mucosal lining of the inner cheek
Canth/o (CAN-tho)	The corners of the eyes, literally meaning "slanted"	Canthoplasty, a surgical procedure to adjust the outer corners of the eyelids
Capit/o (CAP-it-oh)	The head, or head-like	Decapitation, removal of the head, usually due to trauma
Carp/o (CARP-oh)	Wrist	Carpal tunnel, the narrow passageway for tendons and nerves in the wrist
Caud/o (CAW-do)	Tail	Caudad, in the direction of or toward the tail
Cephal/o (SEFF-ah-lo)	Head	Cephalad, in the direction of or toward the head
Cervic/o (SIR-vick-oh)	Neck	Cervicalgia, neck pain

EXTERNAL ROOT WORDS		
ROOT WORD	MEANING	EXAMPLE
Cheil/o (KAI-lo)	Lips	Cheiloplasty, surgical lip restoration
Faci/o (FACE-ee-oh)	Face	Facioplegia, paralysis of the face muscles
Gingiv/o (GIN-jih-voh)	Gums	Gingival hyperplasia, an overgrowth of gum tissue
Gloss/o (GLOSS-oh)	Tongue (Greek)	Macroglossia, an abnormally enlarged tongue
Gnath/o (NATHE-oh)	Jaw	Gnathoplasty, surgical reconstruction of the jaw
Inguin/o (INN-gwin-oh)	Groin	Inguinodynia, chronic pain or discomfort of the groin region
Irid/o (ih-RID-oh)	Iris, the colored part of the eye	Iridodonesis, an abnormal condition where the iris vibrates during eye movements
Kine- (KIN or KINE)	Movement	Kinesiology, the study of movement
Labi/a (LAY-bee-uh)	Lips (oral or vaginal)	Labiaplasty, surgical modification of the vagina
Ling/o (LING-oh), **Lingu/o** (LING-you-lo)	Tongue (Latin)	Sublingual, medication that is absorbed under the tongue
Mamm/o (MAM, like Ma'am)	Breast (Latin)	Mammogram, a radiographic image of the breasts to identify cancerous tumors
Mast/o (MAST-oh)	Breast (Greek)	Mastitis, inflammation of the breast; often due to infection
Nas/o (NAZE-oh)	Nose (Latin)	Nasopharynx, where the nose meets the posterior pharynx

(continued)

(continued from previous page)

EXTERNAL ROOT WORDS		
ROOT WORD	MEANING	EXAMPLE
Occipit/o (ock-SIP-it-oh)	Back of head	Occipital lobe, the brain region located at the back of the head
Ocul/o (OCK-you-lo)	Eye	Oculomotor nerve, the cranial nerve that controls most eye movement muscles
Odont/o (oh-DAHNT-oh)	Tooth, teeth	Odontogenic infection, an infection that originates in the teeth
Omphal/o (om-FAL-oh)	Belly button, navel (Greek)	Omphalocele, a birth anomaly in which the infant's intestines protrude out of the body
Onych/o (ON-ick-oh)	Relating to nails	Onychomycosis, a fungal infection of the nails, most commonly toenails
Ophthalm/o (opp-THAL-mo)	Eye	Ophthalmoscope, an instrument for inspecting the eye
Opt/o (OPT-oh)	Eye, vision	Optometrist, an eye doctor who does not perform surgical procedures
Or/o (OR-oh)	The mouth	Oropharynx, the region of the oral cavity and pharynx
Ot/o (OH-to)	Ear	Otitis media, a middle ear infection
Papill/o (pap-ILL-oh)	Nipple or resembling a nipple	Papillary muscles, the nipple-shaped muscles located in the heart ventricles
Pector (peck-TORR-oh)	Breast or chest	Pectoralis, the major chest muscles
Pelv/o (PELL-vo)	Pelvis or pelvic region	Pelvic floor, muscles located between the tailbone and the pubic bone
Perine/o (per-ih-NEE-oh)	The area between the anus and the scrotum or vulva	Perineorrhaphy, suturing or repair of the perineum

EXTERNAL ROOT WORDS		
ROOT WORD	MEANING	EXAMPLE
Phall/o (FA-lo)	Phallus, penis	Phalloplasty, surgical construction or reconstruction of a penis
Pil/o (PIE-lo)	Relating to hair, or hair-like structures	Piloerection, when hair stands on end, also known as "goosebumps"
Pod/o (PO-doh)	Foot	Podiatrist, a surgeon who specializes in the foot, ankle, and lower leg
Rhin/o (RYE-no)	Relating to the nose	Rhinoplasty, surgical augmentation of the nose
Somat/o (so-MAT-oh)	Body, bodily	Somatic nerves, nerves that control the body's voluntary movement
Steth/o (STETH-oh)	Chest	Stethoscope, a device used to auscultate (listen to) the body, particularly to the chest
Stomat/o (sto-MAT-oh)	Mouth	Stomatitis, inflammation of the lips and mouth
Tal/o (TAIL-oh)	Ankle	Talocrural joint, the ankle joint
Tars/o (TAR-so)	Ankle/foot	Metatarsals, the long bones of the feet
Thorac/o (thorr-ACK-oh)	Chest	Thoracotomy, surgical opening of the chest
Trache/o (TRAY-kee-oh)	Relating to the trachea, the first and largest airway portion	Tracheostomy, a surgical procedure in which a hole is placed in the trachea to allow for breathing
Trich/o (TRICK-oh)	Relating to hair	Trichotillomania, a psychological condition in which a person has irresistible urges to pull out their own hair

INTERNAL ROOT WORDS

The following table outlines some key root words that relate to internal body structures but don't fit neatly into the organ systems we previously listed. That doesn't mean they're not important. I use many of these terms daily.

INTERNAL ROOT WORDS		
ROOT WORD	MEANING	EXAMPLE
Acou (ah-KOO)	Relating to hearing	Hyperacusis, a heightened sense of hearing
Aer/o (AIR-oh)	Air, gas	Aerophagia, swallowing air
Alge (al-GEE), **Algi/o** (al-GEE-oh)	Pain	Analgesic, a drug or treatment to relieve pain
Bacillus (bas-ILL-us)	Rod-shaped	Bacillus, a rod-shaped bacterium
Bacter/i (back-TEER-ee)	Pertaining to bacteria	Bacteremia, bacteria in the bloodstream
Blast (BLAST)	Create, originate	Osteoblast, a cell that creates bone
Carcin/o (car-SIN-oh)	Cancer	Carcinogen, a substance known to cause cancer
Cellul/o (CELL-you-lo)	Cells	Cellular membrane, the outer layer of a cell
Cholecyst/o (koll-ee-SIS-to)	Gallbladder	Cholecystitis, inflammation of the gallbladder
Cili/o (SIH-lee-oh)	Hair-like, or relating to the ciliary muscle of the eye	Ciliary dyskinesia, improper function of the hair-like cilia that line the respiratory tract
Cortic/o (core-TIC-oh)	Cortex, outer region	Renal cortex, the outer region of the kidney
Cost/o (COST-oh)	Ribs and ribcage	Costochondritis, inflammation of the ribs

INTERNAL ROOT WORDS		
ROOT WORD	MEANING	EXAMPLE
Cry/o (CRY-oh)	Cold	Cryoablation, using cold instruments to ablate, or damage, tissue
Crypt/o (KRIPT-oh)	Hidden, secret	Cryptogenic, a disease of obscure or uncertain origin
Cyt/o (SITE-oh)	Cells	Cytology, the study of cells
Enter/o (EN-ter-oh)	Any part of the small intestine	Enterovirus, a viral pathogen affecting the small intestine
Episi/o (epp-EASY-oh)	Vulva, the external female genitalia	Episiotomy, a tear in the vagina during childbirth
Fibr/o (FYE-bro)	Fibers, scar tissue	Fibrosis, the process of thickening of tissue into a scar
Foramen, Foramin (fore-AY-min)	A hole or opening, often in bone	Foramen magnum, the large hole at the skull base through which the brainstem passes
Fossa (FOSS-ah)	A hollow or depressed area	Supraclavicular fossa, the small depressions above the collarbones
Galact/o (guh-LACT-oh)	Milk	Galactorrhea, milk flowing out of nipples other than during breast feeding
Gon/i (GO-nee)	Seed, reproduction	Gonads, organs that produce gametes (sperm or eggs)
Hemat/o (he-MAT-oh)	Blood	Hematology, the study of blood disorders
Hist/o (HISS-toe)	Tissue	Histology, the study of tissues
Hydr/o (HI-dro)	Water, fluid	Hydrocephalus, abnormal buildup of fluid in the brain
Kal (KALE)	Potassium, from the Greek word "kalium"	Hyperkalemia, high blood potassium levels
Lact/o (LACK-toe)	Milk	Lactation, milk production

(continued)

(*continued from previous page*)

INTERNAL ROOT WORDS

ROOT WORD	MEANING	EXAMPLE
Lapar/o (LAP-ar-oh)	Abdominal wall	Laparoscopy, minimally invasive surgery of the abdomen
Lith/o (LITH-oh)	Stone	Nephrolithiasis, the presence of kidney stones
Nat/o (NATE-oh)	Birth	Prenatal, before birth
Necr/o (NECK-ro)	Death	Necrosis, death of body tissue
Onc/o (ONK-oh)	Tumor, cancer	Oncology, the specialty of cancer diagnosis and treatment
Phos (FOSS)	Phosphorous	Hypophosphatemia, low blood phosphorus
Presby (PRESS-bee)	Relating to old age	Presbyopia, natural vision loss that occurs with old age
Pyr/o (PIE-ro)	Fever or heat	Antipyretics, medications to reduce fevers
Sept/o (SEPT-oh)	A dividing wall or membrane	Septoplasty, a surgical procedure to straighten the nasal septum and cartilage
Ser/o (SER-oh)	The clear liquid part of blood or the slippery lining of internal organs	Serositis, inflammation of "serous" tissues of the body including the peritoneum, pericardium, and pleura
Terat/o (TERR-at-oh)	Literally "monster," or unusual in appearance	Teratogen, a substance that causes birth anomalies
Tetan/o (TET-an-oh)	Rigid, tense	Tetanus, a state of severe muscle contraction
Therm/o (THERR-mo)	Heat or temperature	Hypothermia, abnormally low body temperature
Thromb/o (THROM-bo)	Blood clot or clotting; platelets (which assist in clotting)	Thrombectomy, a surgical procedure to break down and remove a blood clot

DIRECTIONAL ROOT WORDS

In medical practice, it is critical to precisely describe direction and position. Imagine your mentor is helping you perform a bronchoscopy, a procedure in which a small flexible camera is used to examine the lungs. You would need to precisely understand your colleague's instruction regarding direction and position as you maneuvered throughout the airways. The following table lists the key terms that enable this:

- To understand the terms "ventral" and "dorsal," imagine the human body walking on all fours. The dorsal surfaces are those where sun would naturally shine, including the back of your hands and the tops of the feet. Ventral surfaces remain in the shade.

- "Cranial" means toward the head and "caudal" means toward the tail, but I recommend using the terms "superior" and "inferior," respectively, as they are more precise.

- You can use the connecting "o" to link these terms for more specificity. For instance, "anterolateral" for "anterior and lateral."

DIRECTIONAL ROOT WORDS		
ROOT WORD	MEANING	EXAMPLE
Anterior	Toward the front of the body	The breastbone is anterior to the heart.
Ventral		The belly button is located on the ventral body surface.
Caudal	Below, lower, or "toward the tailbone"	The lumbar spine is caudal to the thoracic spine.
Inferior		The toes are inferior to the knees.
Cranial	Above, higher, or "toward the head"	The shoulders are cranial to the hips.
Superior		The eyelids are superior to the lips.

(continued)

(continued from previous page)

DIRECTIONAL ROOT WORDS		
ROOT WORD	MEANING	EXAMPLE
Deep	Farther away from the surface, or closer to the absolute center of the body	The hypodermis is deep compared to the epidermis.
Distal	Further away from the spine; often referring to structures of the limbs	The wrist is distal to the elbow.
Dorsal	Toward the back of the body	The spine is dorsal to the abdomen.
Posterior		The esophagus is posterior to the heart.
External	Outside or outer	The skin is external to the internal organs.
Internal	Inside or inner	The heart is internal to the ribcage.
Lateral	Away from the midline (from the sagittal plane)	The shoulders are lateral to the breastbone.
Medial	Toward the midline (from the sagittal plane)	The nose is medial to the eyes.
Palmar	The palm side of the hand	Some rashes occur only on the palmar surface of the hands.
Plantar	The sole side of the foot (the side that is touching the ground when standing)	Plantar warts occur on the bottoms of the feet.
Proximal	Closer to the axial skeleton; often referring to structures of the limbs	The elbow is proximal to the wrist.
Superficial	Closer to the surface	The skin is superficial to the muscles.
Valgus	Turned inward	In "knock knees," the knees have a valgus deformity, also known as "genu" (knee) valgum.

DIRECTIONAL ROOT WORDS		
ROOT WORD	MEANING	EXAMPLE
Varus	Turned outward	When someone is "bowlegged," the knees are in a varus deformity, also known as "genu" varum.

COMBINING ROOT WORDS WITH SUFFIXES AND PREFIXES

Congratulations on learning the vast majority of medical root words! You are now ready to dive into prefixes and suffixes. This is where the real fun begins. Most often, you will simply stick the prefix in front of the root, or the suffix after the root. However, you will need to pay some attention to the letters that join them. In general, medical terms avoid linking more than two vowels together. If this is the case, one vowel will often be dropped to make the term flow better. In the next chapters, pay attention to where the connecting "o" is used and where it is omitted. Let's look at a few examples.

Cardi (root) + -ology (suffix) = Cardiology (not "cardioology")

Hyper- (prefix) + glyc (root) + -emia (suffix) = Hyperglycemia
(not hyperglycoemia, unless you're in the United Kingdom
where they have different spelling conventions)

Hemato (root) + -poiesis (suffix, "to produce") = Hematopoiesis
(notice the "o" is included)

If you create a medical term that sounds clunky when spoken, try adding or removing the connecting "o."

KEY TAKEAWAYS

This chapter concluded our study of root words. We covered terms for external and internal body parts that otherwise do not neatly fit into the standard organ systems. We also learned key directional and positional terms. Here are the key takeaways from this chapter:

- The terms "dorsal" and "ventral" are best visualized by imagining humans walking on all fours.

- The terms "superior" and "inferior" are preferred over "cranial" and "caudal" because they are more specific and universal.

- When linking roots with prefixes and suffixes, be mindful of the connecting "o," and avoid situations where more than two vowels are joined side-by-side.

Now you are ready to learn how to add prefixes and suffixes to these roots, which will allow you to create thousands of medical terms. But first, let's test your memory of the terms we learned in this chapter.

1. The term "gingivitis" refers to inflammation of the _____.

   a. gums

   b. meninges

   c. gallbladder

2. What does the term "cholelithiasis" refer to?

   a. kidney stones

   b. gallstones

   c. gallbladder surgery

3. The eyes are superior and _____ to the nose.

   a. medial

   b. caudal

   c. lateral

4. The soles of the feet are on the _____ surface, also known as "plantar."

   a. ventral

   b. dorsal

5. The knees are _____ to the feet.

   a. superior

   b. inferior

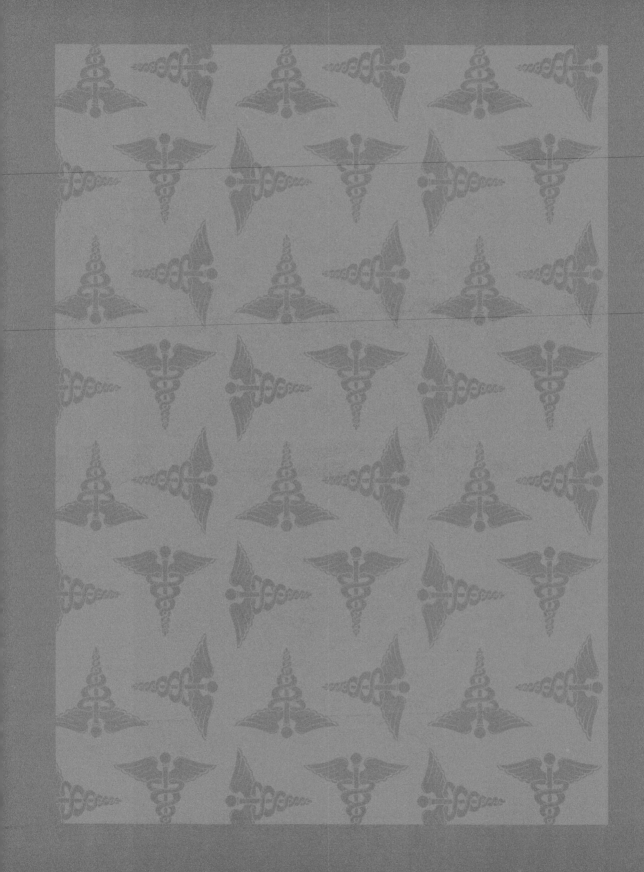

CHAPTER 5

PREFIXES

A s I mentioned in part 1, a prefix is added to the beginning of a word to alter the root. Classically, prefixes can indicate position, direction, quantity, color, size, or character. But practically speaking, a prefix can indicate almost anything.

The familiar term "disease" is a perfect example of a prefix that dramatically alters the word. The prefix "dis" means "to separate from," so the term "disease" refers to a state of being separated from "ease," or comfort. In this case, adding the prefix transforms the root into its opposite.

You will often see root words used as prefixes as well. For example, the word "*myo*carditis" (heart muscle inflammation) has the prefix "myo," a root word meaning "muscle." It indicates inflammation that occurs in the heart muscle. Fortunately, you are already familiar with many of the roots that get used as prefixes.

This chapter begins with the most commonly occurring prefixes. Then you'll learn prefixes in groups relating to position, direction, number, measurement, color, and characteristics. As you work your way through this chapter, seeing prefixes added to the roots that you've learned, I believe you'll really deepen your understanding of how medical terms are constructed.

TECHNIQUES FOR LEARNING AND RECOGNIZING PREFIXES

It's easy to recognize a prefix; simply look at the first letter or first few letters of a term. It's even easier if you first identify the root word and then focus on any syllables in front of it. Once you master this chapter's prefixes, they will become even easier to identify.

Flash cards are your best friends for efficiently practicing and mastering this material. Review the examples in this chapter and complete the quiz at the end to best help you retain the information. There are admittedly quite a few prefixes to learn, but the effort will be worth it; these prefixes are extremely useful for understanding medical terminology. Once you master this chapter, you will have passed the halfway point, with only suffixes to learn (and some nonstandard terminology that we'll cover in the final chapter).

PREFIXES PERTAINING TO POSITION AND DIRECTION

As we discussed in chapter 2, medical terms to describe body position and direction are integral to the medical language. As with roots, there are many key prefixes that describe position and direction.

POSITION AND DIRECTION PREFIXES		
PREFIX	MEANING	EXAMPLE
Ab-, Abs- (AB)	Away from	Abduction, moving arms or legs away from the sagittal plane
Ad- (ADD)	Toward	Adductors, the muscles that help bring the legs together

POSITION AND DIRECTION PREFIXES		
PREFIX	MEANING	EXAMPLE
Ana- (AN-uh)	Back, against	Anaplastic, when cancer cells mutate and bear no resemblance to their original type
Ante- (ANT-ee)	Before, in front of	Antepartum, the time before delivery
Ap/o- (AY-po)	Next to, nearby	Apposition, placing two objects next to each other
Circum- (sir-COME)	Around (the perimeter)	Circumscribed, when a rash or skin lesion has a well-defined border
Dextr/o- (DEX-trow)	Right, rightward	Dextrocardia, when the heart is positioned on the right side of the chest
Di- (DYE)	Separate, apart	Pupil dilation, the widening of the pupils
Dia- (DYE-ah)	Through or across	Dialysis, filtering blood to correct electrolyte imbalances and remove toxins
Ec- (ECK)	Out, away	Ectopic pregnancy, when a fetus implants outside of the uterus
Ecto- (ECK-toe)	Outside	Ectoderm, the outermost layers of cells in an embryo
En-, **Endo-** (EN-doh)	Inside, within	Endovascular, a procedure that occurs within blood vessels

(continued)

(*continued from previous page*)

POSITION AND DIRECTION PREFIXES

PREFIX	MEANING	EXAMPLE
Epi- (EP-ee)	On, upon	Epicardial, on the outside of the heart
Ex-, Extra- (EX-truh)	Outside, beyond	Extracorporeal, occurring outside of the body, as in extracorporeal membranous oxygenation (ECMO)
Exo- (EX-oh)	Outside	Exocrine, chemicals released outside the body or onto the skin
Fore- (FOR)	Before or ahead	Foregut, the first portion of the digestive tract
Infra- (IN-fruh)	Below	Infrarenal, below the renal arteries
Inter- (IN-terr)	Between	Interstitium, a fluid-filled space between body tissues
Intra- (IN-truh)	Within	Intraparenchymal, a lesion or process occurring within the parenchyma (tissue) of an organ
Intus- (IN-tuss)	Within	Intussusception, when a portion of intestine gets stuck inside of itself
Ipsi- (IP-sih or IP-see)	Same	Ipsilateral, on the same side
Kyph/o- (KAI-foh)	Excessive forward leaning of the thoracic spine	Kyphotic, excessive forward bending of the spine
Lord/o- (LORD-oh)	Excessive inward leaning of the lumbar spine	Lordotic, exaggerated lumbar spine curvature
Meso- (ME-zoh)	Middle	Mesoderm, the middle layers of cells in an embryo

POSITION AND DIRECTION PREFIXES		
PREFIX	MEANING	EXAMPLE
Para- (PAIR-uh)	Alongside, beside, nearby	Paracrine, signal molecules secreted locally, not carried in the bloodstream
Path/o- (PATH-oh)	Disease	Pathophysiology, the study of disease and its effects on physiology
Per- (PER)	Through	Percutaneous, through the skin
Peri- (PER-ee)	Around	Pericardium, the durable sac that surrounds the heart
Post- (POST)	After, behind	Postoperative, after a surgery has been performed
Pre- (PRE)	In front of, before	Preprandial, before meals
Pro- (PRO)	In front of, before	Prodrome, a sense that something is about to occur or an early symptom of a disease
Retro- (RET-row)	Backward, behind	Retrocardiac, behind the heart
Sinistr/o- (SIN-iss-trow)	Left, left-sided	Sinistrocardia, the displacement of the heart to the left
Sub- (SUB)	Under, below, less	Subcutaneous, just below the epidermis and dermis
Super- (SOUP-er), **Supra-** (SOUP-ruh)	Above, upper, over	Supraglottic, the portion of the voice box above the glottis
Trans- (TRANS)	Across, opposite	Transcranial magnetic stimulation, a brain stimulation sending magnetic fields across the skull

PREFIXES PERTAINING TO NUMBER AND MEASUREMENT

I hope that by now, learning new medical terms feels natural to you. Even if that's not the case, you'll find yourself on familiar ground with some of the prefixes in this next batch. For example, you probably already know that the prefix "bi" relates to the number two, as in the two wheels of a *bi*cycle or the two centuries of a *bi*centennial. Keep alert for other well-known instances in the following table of prefixes relating to number and measurement. These are frequently encountered in clinical practice.

NUMBER AND MEASUREMENT PREFIXES		
PREFIX	MEANING	EXAMPLE
Bi- (BYE)	Two	Bilateral, both sides
Di- (DYE)	Two, twice, double	Diplopia, double vision
Hemi- (HEM-ee)	Half	Hemiplegia, weakness of half of the body (left or right)
Iso- (EYE-so)	Equal, equivalent	Isotonic, two solutions with the same tonicity
Mon/o- (MON)	Single, one	Monocular, one eye
Nulli- (NULL-ee)	None, zero	Nulliparous, having never given birth
Olig/o- (oh-LIG-oh)	Few, scant, little	Oliguria, decreased urine output
Pauci- (PAW-see)	Few, small, scant	Pauci-immune, a type of renal injury with very few immunoglobulins seen on microscopy
Pleio- (PLEE-oh)	More, excessive	Pleocytosis, an increased cell count in a bodily fluid
Poly- (POLL-ee)	Many, much, excessive	Polyuria, excessive urination
Prim/i- (PRIM-ee)	One, first	Primigravida, first pregnancy

NUMBER AND MEASUREMENT PREFIXES		
PREFIX	MEANING	EXAMPLE
Quadri- (QUAD-rih)	Four	Quadriceps, the four large thigh muscles
Semi- (SEM-ee)	Half	Semiconscious, not fully alert
Tetra- (TET-ruh)	Four	Tetraplegia, paralysis of all four extremities, also called "quadriplegia"
Tri- (TRI)	Three	Triceps, the posterior upper arm muscle that has three "heads" or insertion sites
Uni- (YOU-nee)	One	Unilateral, involving only one side

The metric system is used in health care throughout the world, so knowing metric prefixes is critical—especially in the case of dosages.

METRIC PREFIXES	
PREFIX	MEANING
Pico-	One trillionth (10^{-12})
Nano-	One billionth (10^{-9})
Micro-	One millionth (10^{-6})
Milli-	One thousandth (10^{-3})
Centi-	One hundredth (10^{-2})
Deci-	One tenth (10^{-1})
Deka-	Ten (10)
Hecto-	Hundred (10^{2})
Kilo-	Thousand (10^{3})
Mega-	Million (10^{6})
Giga-	Billion (10^{9})
Tera-	Trillion (10^{12})

PREFIXES PERTAINING TO COLOR

Many medical terms describe colors because direct visualization has been, and continues to be, an important part of practicing medicine. In fact, study this list of prefixes describing various colors, and you'll get a sense of how important color can be in identifying a disease or condition.

PREFIXES PERTAINING TO COLOR		
TERM	MEANING	EXAMPLE
Alb/o- (AL-bo), **Albin/o-** (ael-BINE-oh), **Leuk/o-** (LUKE-oh)	White	Albinism, a group of inherited disorders characterized by a lack of melanin Leukocyte, a white blood cell
Chlor/o- (KLORR-oh)	Green	Chloride, a common electrolyte named after the greenish color of chlorine gas
Cyan/o- (sigh-ANN-oh)	Blue	Cyanosis, blue discoloration, often due to low blood oxygen
Eosin/o- (ee-oh-SIN-oh)	Pink	Eosinophil, immune cells that appear pink on microscopy because they bind tightly to the dye "eosin" which has a pink color
Erythr/o- (eh-RITH-ro), **Rubr/o-** (ROO-bro)	Red	Erythroderma, "red skin" caused by a variety of conditions. Rubrospinal, a nerve tract that controls movement; it arises from the "red nucleus"
Glauc/o- (GLAU-ko)	Gray or blueish	Glaucoma, eye conditions that damage the optic nerve, causing it to appear gray
Melan/o- (meh-LAN-oh), **Nigr/o-** (NYE-gro)	Black	Melanoma, a malignant skin cancer of melanocytes, cells with dark pigment Substantia nigra, the part of the brain that controls fine movements, which appears black due to an abundance of pigment
Purpur/o- (pur-PUR-oh)	Purple	Purpura, a rash of purple spots due to disruption of small blood vessels

PREFIXES PERTAINING TO COLOR		
TERM	MEANING	EXAMPLE
Cirrh/o- (SIR-oh), **Jaund/o-** (JAWN-do), **Xanth/o-** (ZANTH-oh)	Yellow	Cirrhosis, end-stage liver disease which often leads to a yellowing of the skin, called jaundice Xanthochromia, yellow-tinged cerebrospinal fluid

OTHER COMMON PREFIXES

The following prefixes do not neatly fit into the previous categories, but they're very often used in clinical practice.

OTHER COMMON PREFIXES		
PREFIX	MEANING	EXAMPLE
A-, an-	Without, missing, "not"	Asplenia, lacking a spleen
Acanth- (ay-CANTH)	Thorn or spine	Acanthocyte, a red blood cell with a thorn-like projection
All/o- (AL-oh)	Other	Allotransplant, transplantation of an organ or tissue from one person to another
Ambi- (am-BEE)	Both sides, two-sided	Ambidextrous, the ability to use both sides of the body equally
Aniso- (ann-EYE-so)	Describing something as unequal	Anisocoria, pupils of unequal size
Anti- (ANT-ee)	Opposite, against	Antibiotics, medications that work against bacteria
Apo- (AP-oh)	Away or separated from	Apoptosis, programmed cell death
Auto- (AW-toe)	Self	Autoimmune, when the body's immune system attacks itself

(continued)

(continued from previous page)

OTHER COMMON PREFIXES		
PREFIX	MEANING	EXAMPLE
Bovine- (BO-vine)	Resembling or related to cows	Bovine insulin, insulin produced by cow pancreas cells
Brachy- (BRAKE-ee)	Short, little, or small	Brachycephalic, small head
Brady- (BRAY-dee)	Slow	Bradycardia, slow heart rate
Cata- (CAT-uh)	Down, across, under	Cataplexy, a sudden loss of muscle tone leading to collapse
Chem/o- (KEEM-oh)	Chemistry, drug	Chemotherapy, use of chemicals to kill cancer cells
Cis- (SIS)	Same	Cisgender, a person whose gender identification corresponds to their sex assigned at birth
Co-, Con-, Com-	With, together	Contract (an illness), to become ill with a transmissible disease
Contra- (KON-truh)	Against, contrary to, contrasting	Contraindication, a reason to not take a medical treatment due to harm that it may cause
Crypto- (KRIP-toe)	Hidden, secret	Cryptogenic, a disease of obscure or uncertain origin
De- (DEE)	Away from, opposite, ending	Dehydration, to be without or lacking water
Dis- (DIS)	Apart, separated from natural state	Disease, separated from ease or comfort
Dys- (DIS)	Hard, difficult, bad	Dyspnea, difficulty breathing
Hydr/o- (HI-dro)	Water (or water-like liquid)	Hydrocephalus, a buildup of cerebrospinal fluid in the brain
Hyper- (HIPE-rr)	Excessive, above	Hypertension, blood pressure above the normal range
Hypo- (HIPE-oh)	Lacking, below, under	Hypoglycemia, blood glucose below the normal range

OTHER COMMON PREFIXES		
PREFIX	MEANING	EXAMPLE
Iatr/o- (eye-AT-ro)	Healer, healing	Iatrogenic, produced or caused by the medical team
Idio- (ih-DEE-oh)	Distinctive, peculiar to	Idiopathic, a disease or condition of unknown or unexplainable cause. ("It makes us feel like idiots")
Isch- (ISH)	Restriction, restricted	Ischemia, restricted blood flow causing tissue death
Kary- (CARRY)	Nucleus	Karyotype, direct visualization of chromosomes (found in the cell nucleus)
Lei/o- (LIE-oh)	Smooth	Leiomyoma, a benign uterine smooth muscle tumor
Lept/o- (LEPT-oh)	Thin, light, slender	Leptomeningeal, the innermost, thinnest, and most delicate layers of the meninges
Macro- (MACK-ro)	Large	Macrocytosis, red blood cells growing larger than normal
Mega- (MEG-uh)	Very large	Megakaryocyte, a young blood cell that's much larger than other blood cells
Meta- (MET-uh)	Change	Metaplasia, transformation from one cell type to another
Micro- (MIKE-ro)	Tiny	Microscopic, too small to be seen by the naked eye
Myc/o- (MICE or MY-ko)	Fungus	Mycetoma, a collection of fungus, or "fungal ball"
Myx/o- (MIX-oh)	Mucus	Myxoma, a collection of mucus tissue
Narc/o- (NARK-oh)	Numb, sleep	Narcotics, medications known for inducing numbness and sleep

(continued)

(continued from previous page)

OTHER COMMON PREFIXES		
PREFIX	MEANING	EXAMPLE
Neo- (NEE-oh)	New	Neonate, a newborn baby
Nodul/o- (NOD-you-lo)	A round mass	Pulmonary nodule, a round mass in the lungs
Norm/o- (NORM-oh)	"Normal" or expected	Normoxia, normal or appropriate blood oxygen levels
Odyn/o- (oh-DINE-oh)	Painful	Odynophagia, pain with swallowing
Orth/o- (OR-tho)	Straight, in-line, or correct	Orthostatic, an upright posture
Oxy- (OX-ee)	Sharp, acute, keen; oxygen	Oxytocin, a hormone that acutely enhances contractions during labor
Pachy- (PACK-ee)	Thick	Pachycephaly, an abnormally thick skull
Pan-	All or everywhere	Pancytopenia, a reduction in all three major blood cell lineages
Pharmaco- (FARM-uh-ko)	Drug; medicine	Pharmacokinetics, how the body metabolizes and eliminates medications
Porcine- (POUR-seen)	Resembling or related to pigs	Porcine valve, a heart valve created with pig tissue
Pseud/o- (SUE-doe)	Fake or false	Pseudohyponatremia, falsely low sodium due to an error in measurement
Py/o- (PIE-oh)	Pus	Pyogenic, producing pus
Re-	Again, backward	Rejuvenation, giving new energy or vigor

OTHER COMMON PREFIXES		
PREFIX	MEANING	EXAMPLE
Reticul/o- (re-TICK-you-lo)	Net	Reticular pattern, a net-like appearance, often used to describe chest x-ray findings
Sanguin- (san-GWIN)	Blood	Sanguinous, fluid containing blood
Scoli/o- (sko-LEE-oh)	Twisted	Scoliosis, a sideways curvature of the spine
Somat/o- (so-MAH-to), **Somatic/o-** (so-mah-TICK-oh)	Body, bodily	Somatic nerves, nerves that control the body's voluntary movement
Stomat/o- (sto-MAH-to)	Mouth	Stomatitis, inflammation of the lips and mouth
Syn- (SIN), **Sym-** (SIM)	Together, combining	Synesthesia, the mixing of sensory information
Tachy- (TACK-ee)	Fast	Tachycardia, a fast heart rate
Trans- (TRANS)	Across	Transthoracic echocardiogram, a heart ultrasound obtained by transmitting sound waves across the chest wall
Ultra- (ULL-truh)	Extreme, beyond	Ultraviolet, radiation with a wavelength beyond the spectrum of visible light
Xeno- (ZEE-no)	Stranger or "other"	Xenotransplantation, transplanting organs, tissues, or cells from one species to another
Xer/o- (ZERO)	Dry	Xerostomia, dry mouth

PREFIX ANTONYMS

Some medical terms are antonyms, or words that mean the opposite of each other. This table presents important antonym pairings. There are two instances in which there are a trio of terms because multiple words are commonly used.

PREFIX ANTONYMS		
PREFIX	MEANING	EXAMPLE
Ab-, Abs- (Ab)	Away from, apart	Abduction, to move away from the sagittal plane
Ad- (Ad)	To, toward, near	Adduction, to move toward the sagittal plane
Allo- (AL-o)	Other	Allotransplant, transplantation of an organ or tissue from one person to another
Auto- (AW-toe)	Self	Autoimmune, when the body's immune system attacks itself
Andr/o- (AN-dro)	Male	Androgens, male sex hormones, classically testosterone
Gyn/o- (GINE), **Gynec/o-** (gy-NEC-oh)	Women, female	Gynecologist, a doctor who specializes in women's health, particularly of the reproductive organs
Anter/o- (ANN-ter-oh)	Front, in front of	Anterolisthesis, when a vertebral body slips forward in relation to the one below
Poster/o- (POSS-ter-oh)	Behind, in back of	Posterior chamber, the portion of the eye behind the lens
Retr/o- (RET-ro)	Behind, backward	Retrocardiac, behind the heart
Bio- (BY-oh)	Life	Biology, the study of life and living things

PREFIX ANTONYMS		
PREFIX	MEANING	EXAMPLE
Necr/o- (NECK-ro)	Death	Necrosis, death of body tissue
Brady- (BRAY-dee)	Slow	Bradycardia, slow heart rate
Tachy- (TACK-ee)	Fast	Tachycardia, fast heart rate
Cis- (SIS)	Same	Cisgender, a person whose gender identity corresponds to their sex assigned at birth
Trans- (TRANS)	Across	Transthoracic echocardiogram, a heart ultrasound obtained by transmitting sound waves across the chest wall
Dys- (DIS)	Difficult, abnormal	Dyspnea, labored breathing
Mal- (MAL)	Bad, abnormal	Malignant, cancerous
Eu- (YOU)	Good, well	Eupnea, breathing comfortably
Endo- (EN-doh)	Within	Endocrine, hormones secreted within the bloodstream
Exo- (EX-oh)	Outside	Exocrine, chemicals released outside of the body or to the skin
Hetero- (HET-er-oh)	Other, different	Heterozygous, having two different alleles of a gene
Homo- (HO-mo)	Same	Homozygous, having two identical alleles of a gene
Hyper- (HIPE-err)	Excessive, above	Hypertension, blood pressure above the normal range
Hypo- (HIPE-oh)	Lacking, below, under	Hypoglycemia, blood glucose below the normal range
Later/o- (LAT-er-oh)	To the side	Lateral meniscus, the outside band in the knee joint
Medi/o- (ME-dee-oh)	Toward the midline	Medial meniscus, the inner band in the knee joint

PREFIX SYNONYMS

You have already encountered a few examples of medical terms in which both Greek and Latin versions are commonly used. It is important to be aware of these since you might encounter either, depending on the situation. The following table presents common Greek and Latin synonyms.

PREFIX SYNONYMS		
MEANING	GREEK	LATIN
Bad	Dys-	Mal-
Breast	Mast/o-	Mamm/o-
Fingernail	Onych/o-	Ungu/o-
Hair	Trich/o-	Pil/o-
Head	Cephal/o-	Crani/o-
Kidneys	Nephr/o-	Ren/o-
Navel (Belly Button)	Omphal/o-	Umbilic/o-
Nose	Rhin/o-	Nas/o-
Ovary	Oophor/o-	Ovari/o-
Testes	Orch/o-, Orchi/o-	Test/o-, Testicul/o-
Tongue	Gloss/o-	Ling/o-, Lingul/o-
Tooth	Odont/o-	Dent/o-
Uterus	Hyster/o-, Metr/o-	Uter/o-
Vagina	Colp/o-	Vagin/o-
Vein	Phleb-	Vein/o-

KEY TAKEAWAYS

Congratulations on completing another chapter jam-packed with important medical terminology! You've now learned virtually every prefix you will encounter in medicine. Now that you know roots and prefixes, it's time to look at medical suffixes. But first, here are the key takeaways from this chapter:

- Prefixes are the first letter or first few letters of a term that precede the root word.

- Prefixes often describe colors, numbers or quantity, or bodily position or direction. However, many don't fit into those categories and indicate other meanings.

- Some prefixes have opposite meanings and can be used to create words that are antonyms of each other.

- Many Greek and Latin prefixes have identical meanings, and it is important to be able to use both.

1. Pancytopenia refers to a reduction in _____.
   a. red blood cells only
   b. platelets only
   c. white blood cells only
   d. all of the major blood cell lineages

2. The medical term for "normal breathing" is _____.
   a. dyspnea
   b. eupnea
   c. apnea

3. The outside layer of the skin is known as the ___dermis.
   a. meso
   b. endo
   c. epi

4. An *infrarenal* abdominal aortic aneurysm occurs _____ the renal arteries.
   a. above
   b. inside
   c. below

5. Oligoarthritis refers to inflammation in _____ joint(s).
   a. one
   b. a few
   c. every

6. Which of the following measurements is larger?
   a. microgram
   b. milligram

7. Brady means slow and _____ means fast.
   a. hyper
   b. ultra
   c. tachy

8. If you receive a transplant of your own stem cells, it is known as a(n) ___ transplant.
   a. auto
   b. allo
   c. xeno

9. Uter/o is the Latin prefix for uterus, what is the Greek term?
   a. phleb/o
   b. omphal/o
   c. hyster/o

10. An abundance of white blood cells is known as a(n) _____cytosis.
    a. erythro
    b. leuko
    c. glauco
    d. cyano

ANSWERS

1.d   2.b   3.c   4.c   5.b   6.b   7.c   8.a   9.c   10.b

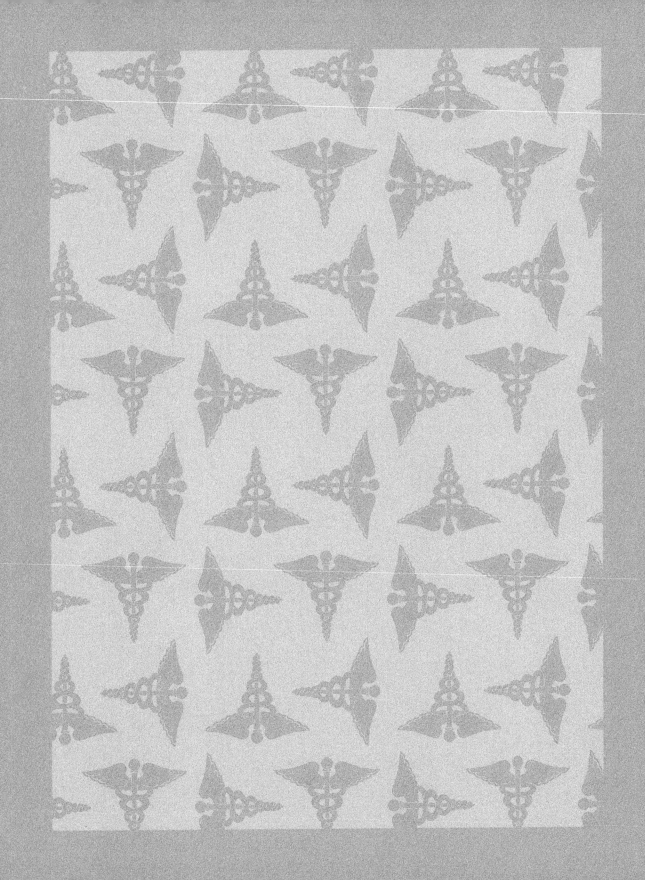

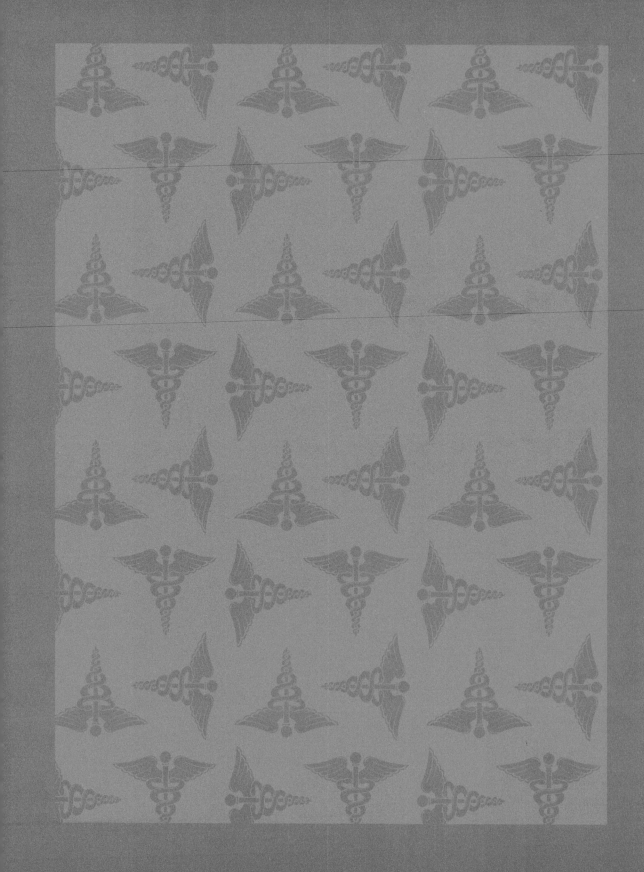

CHAPTER 6

SUFFIXES

This chapter is all about the caboose of medical terms, the suffix. As we discussed earlier, the suffix is the ending of the word and significantly shapes its meaning. Suffixes can indicate everything from orientation to color, shape, category, function, disease, and specialty. In this chapter, we'll review suffixes relating to surgeries and procedures, pathologies or diseases, and medical specialties. You'll also learn grammatical suffixes and some commonly used suffixes that do not fit well into the other categories. Along the way, you will see many familiar roots and prefixes, so this chapter will be a great opportunity to review some of what you've learned so far.

TECHNIQUES FOR LEARNING AND RECOGNIZING SUFFIXES

By now, you're an expert at breaking terms into their component pieces. For this chapter, pay close attention to the last few letters of each term to identify the suffix. Since there is so much information, I recommend you pull out those flash cards to study and retain this material. I also suggest you look for examples of these suffixes in your daily life. Have you ever heard of lactose intolerance, which causes people to be intolerant of dairy products? They lack the enzyme lact*ase* (-ase = enzyme) to digest lact*ose* (-ose = sugar), the dominant sugar in milk. Finding non-medical examples like that will hone your skill at identifying the suffixes within medical terms.

SUFFIXES FOR SURGICAL AND DIAGNOSTIC PROCEDURES

There are many medical terms that describe surgeries and procedures. They are often quite long, for instance, "esophagogastroduodenoscopy." Fortunately, that one is most commonly referred to as an "EGD." Can you deduce the definition of EGD? (If not, the answer is provided at the end of this chapter.) By learning these key suffixes, you will be able to decipher the meaning of many surgeries and procedures.

SUFFIXES FOR SURGICAL AND DIAGNOSTIC PROCEDURES		
SUFFIX	MEANING	EXAMPLE
-centesis (cent-EE-sis)	Surgical puncture to remove fluid	Paracentesis, a procedure in which fluid is removed from the abdomen
-clasis (CLAY-sis)	To break	Osteoclasis, a procedure in which a bone is broken in order to be repaired

SUFFIXES FOR SURGICAL AND DIAGNOSTIC PROCEDURES		
SUFFIX	MEANING	EXAMPLE
-clysis (CLEE-sis)	Irrigating, washing	Hypodermoclysis, a method of infusing fluid into subcutaneous tissue
-crit (KRITT)	To separate	Hematocrit, a blood test that separates blood components
-desis (DEE-sis)	Fusion	Pleurodesis, surgically adhering the lung to the chest wall
-ectomy (ECK-tuh-me)	Surgical removal	Appendectomy, surgical removal of the appendix
-gram (GRAM)	Record or picture	Echocardiogram, a device that uses sound waves to visualize the heart
-graph (GRAFF)	Instrument used to record data or picture	Electrocardiograph, a machine that records the electrical function of the heart
-graphy (GRAFF-ee)	Process of recording	Angiography, a radiographic study or invasive procedure that examines arteries
-meter (ME-ter)	An instrument used to measure or count	Thermometer, an instrument that measures temperature
-metry (MEH-tree)	The process of measuring	Goniometry, measuring the range of motion of a joint
-opsy (OPP-see)	To view	Biopsy, obtaining a sample of tissue to examine it closely

(continued)

(continued from previous page)

SUFFIXES FOR SURGICAL AND DIAGNOSTIC PROCEDURES		
SUFFIX	MEANING	EXAMPLE
-pexy (PEX-ee)	Fixation or attachment	Gastropexy, surgical attachment of the stomach to the abdominal wall
-pheresis (fer-EE-sis)	Removal	Plasmapheresis, a procedure to separate, remove, and replace blood plasma
-plasty (PLAS-ty)	Surgical repair, reconstruction	Rhinoplasty, surgical modification of the nose
-rrhaphy (RAH-fee)	Surgical suturing	Enterorrhaphy, surgically suturing together a hole in the intestine
-scope (SCOPE)	Instrument for viewing	Colonoscope, a long flexible camera used to view the colon
-scopic (SCOPE-ick)	Using small cameras to assist with surgery	Arthroscopic surgery, "keyhole" surgery of a joint
-scopy (SCOPE-ee)	Process of viewing	Endoscopy, a procedure where a long flexible camera is used to view the intestines
-stomy (STO-me)	Creation of an opening	Colostomy, a surgical procedure in which a piece of colon is diverted to an artificial opening in the abdominal wall
-tome (TOME, like "home")	An instrument used to cut	Microtome, a device used to precisely slice tissue
-tripsy (TRIP-see)	Crushing	Sonolithotripsy, using sound waves to crush stones, often kidney stones

SUFFIXES FOR PATHOLOGIES

To an internist like myself, this next table of "pathological condition suffixes" is the real "meat and potatoes" of my medical vocabulary. These suffixes describe a variety of diseases and conditions that I encounter in my medical practice. You'll likely come across these terms, whether you work in health care or are a patient. I know I'm biased, but I suggest spending a little extra time learning these.

SUFFIXES FOR PATHOLOGICAL CONDITIONS		
SUFFIX	MEANING	EXAMPLE
-asthenia (as-THEE-nee-uh)	Weakness	Myasthenia gravis, an autoimmune neurological condition producing skeletal muscle weakness
-atresia (a-TREE-shuh)	A condition in which an orifice or passage does not fully develop	Biliary atresia, when the biliary duct does not form in development
-bilia (bill-EE-uh)	Relating to bile or the biliary tract	Pneumobilia, air in the biliary tract
-carcinoma (car-sin-OH-muh)	Cancer of skin or tissues that line internal organs	Adenocarcinoma, cancer of glandular tissue, often in the colon
-cele (SEAL)	Pouching, hernia	Varicocele, a pouch-like enlargement of the veins within the scrotum
-cidal (SIDE-all), **-cide** (SIDE)	Killing, destroying	Bactericidal, antibiotics that kill bacteria
-clast (KLAST)	To break (down)	Osteoclasts, cells that break down bones
-coccus (KOCK-us)	Round, spherical	Streptococcus, a type of pathogenic bacteria shaped like a sphere

(continued)

(*continued from previous page*)

SUFFIXES FOR PATHOLOGICAL CONDITIONS

SUFFIX	MEANING	EXAMPLE
-dactyly (DACK-till-ee)	Pertaining to a finger or toe	Polydactyly, a condition in which a person has more than 5 fingers or toes on a hand or foot
-dipsia (DIP-see-uh)	Thirst	Polydipsia, excessive thirst
-dynia (DIN-ee-uh)	Pain	Vulvodynia, a chronic pain syndrome of the vulva
-ectasia (eck-TAY-shuh)	Expansion, dilation	Telangiectasia, a condition characterized by dilation of the capillaries
-edema (eh-DEE-ma)	Swelling	Acroedema, swelling of the hands or feet
-emesis (EM-eh-sis)	Vomiting	Hematemesis, vomiting blood
-emia (EE-me-uh)	The presence of a substance in the bloodstream	Uremia, abnormally elevated urea in the bloodstream
-genic (JEN-ick)	Causing, producing, forming	Carcinogenic, cancer-causing
-ia (EE-ah)	Condition of diseased or abnormal state	Bulimia, an eating disorder
-iasis (EYE-ah-sis)	Condition, formation, or presence of	Mydriasis, dilated pupils
-ictal (ICK-tuhl)	Relating to seizures	Postictal, the time after a seizure occurs
-ismus (ISS-mus)	Spasm, contraction	Trismus, lockjaw
-itis (EYE-tis)	Inflammation	Pancreatitis, inflammation of the pancreas
-lith (LITH)	Stone	Cholelith, gallstone
-lysis (LIE-sis)	Destruction, separation	Paralysis, complete or partial loss of strength

SUFFIXES FOR PATHOLOGICAL CONDITIONS		
SUFFIX	MEANING	EXAMPLE
-lytic (LIH-tick)	An agent that attenuates or destroys	Anxiolytic, a medication that reduces anxiety
-malacia (ma-LAY-see-uh)	Softening	Myelomalacia, a softening of the spinal cord due to injury
-mania (MAY-nee-uh)	Extremely elevated mood	Potomania, excessive alcohol consumption
-megaly (MEG-uh-ly)	Irregular enlargement	Cardiomegaly, an enlarged heart
-oma (OH-ma)	Tumor, mass	Mesothelioma, a cancer of the lining of the lungs or abdomen
-orrhage (oh-RAA-gh), **-orrhagia** (oh-RAA-gee-uh)	Excessive flow	Hemorrhage, severe blood loss Menorrhagia, heavy menstruation
-oxia (OX-ee-uh)	Oxygen level	Normoxia, normal blood oxygen concentration
-paresis (PAIR-eh-sis)	Incomplete paralysis, weakness	Hemiparesis, weakness of one side of the body
-pathy (PUH-thy)	Disease or disorder	Retinopathy, disease of the retina
-penia (PEE-nee-uh)	Deficiency	Thrombocytopenia, reduced number of platelets
-phagia (FAY-juh), **-phago** (FAY-go), **-phagy** (FAY-gee)	Swallow, swallowing	Dysphagia, difficulty swallowing
-phasia (FAY-zhuh)	Speech, speaking	Dysphasia, difficulty speaking
-phobia (FO-bee-uh)	exaggerated fear, sensitivity, aversion	Agoraphobia, extreme fear of open or crowded places

(continued)

(continued from previous page)

SUFFIXES FOR PATHOLOGICAL CONDITIONS		
SUFFIX	MEANING	EXAMPLE
-phonia (FO-nee-uh)	Sound, to speak	Aphonia, loss of the ability to speak
-phoria (FOR-ee-uh)	Feeling	Euphoria, a feeling or state of excitement and happiness
-plegia (PLEE-juh)	Paralysis, severe weakness	Tetraplegia, inability to voluntarily move the upper and lower body
-plexy (PLEX-ee)	Sudden change in position	Cataplexy, a sudden loss of muscle tone leading to collapse
-porosis (pour-OH-sis)	Containing many small holes	Osteoporosis, weak and brittle bones
-ptosis (TOH-sis)	Falling, drooping	Apoptosis, programmed cell death Named this because scientists felt it resembled "leaves falling off of a tree"
-ptysis (TISS-iss)	Spitting	Hemoptysis, spitting out blood
-rrhea (REE-uh)	Flow, discharge	Diarrhea, loose watery stools occurring more frequently than normal
-rrhexis (REX-is)	Rupture	Cystorrhexis, rupture of the bladder
-sarcoma (SARK-oh-ma)	Malignant tumor of soft tissues	Chondrosarcoma, a malignant tumor of cartilage cells

SUFFIXES FOR PATHOLOGICAL CONDITIONS		
SUFFIX	MEANING	EXAMPLE
-schisis (SHE-sis)	Separation or cleft	Gastroschisis, a birth anomaly in which the intestines extrude outside of the body
-sclerosis (SKLER-oh-sis)	Hardening	Atherosclerosis, hardening of arteries
-sepsis (SEP-sis)	An overwhelming infection, usually bacterial	Urosepsis, an overwhelming infection from a urinary source
-spadias (SPAY-dee-us)	Slit, fissure	Hypospadias, a birth anomaly in which the urethral opening is positioned below the tip of the penis
-spasm (SPAH-zm)	Spasm, contraction	Bronchospasm, narrowing of the bronchi due to contraction of smooth muscle

SUFFIXES FOR PROFESSIONALS AND SPECIALTIES

Unlike those in the previous table, these suffixes do not necessarily describe diseases. Many of them refer to normal physiology and the medical specialties that concentrate on them.

SUFFIXES FOR PROFESSIONALS AND SPECIALTIES		
SUFFIX	MEANING	EXAMPLE
-acusis (ah-CUE-sis)	Hearing	Presbycusis, hearing loss due to aging
-capnia (CAP-nee-uh)	Carbon dioxide	Hypercapnia, excessive carbon dioxide in the blood

(continued)

(*continued from previous page*)

SUFFIXES FOR PROFESSIONALS AND SPECIALTIES		
SUFFIX	MEANING	EXAMPLE
-cardia (CAR-dee-uh)	Heart	Tachycardia, fast heart rate
-crine (KRINN or KRINE)	Separate, secrete	Endocrine, relating to hormones that are secreted within the bloodstream
-er (ERR)	Operator, a person who performs a procedure	Echocardiographer, the practitioner who performs a heart ultrasound
-iatrics (EE-at-tricks)	Specialty	Pediatrics, medical care for infants, children, and adolescents
-iatry (EYE-uh-tree)	Specialty	Psychiatry, the specialty of mental health
-ician (IH-shun)	A person skilled in a particular subject or activity, specialty	Geriatrician, a physician specializing in the care of elderly patients
-ics (ICKS)	Organized knowledge, specialty	Obstetrics, the study of pregnancy and childbirth
-ist (IST), **-logist** (LO-gist)	A specialist of a particular field	Hospitalist, a doctor who sees patients only in the hospital setting (This is my specialty)
-logy (lo-GEE), **-ology** (AH-lo-gee)	The study or practice of a particular field	Pathology, the study of disease
-opia (OH-pee-uh)	Relating to vision or visual disorders	Myopia, nearsightedness (cannot see far-away objects)
-pepsia (PEP-see-uh)	Relating to digestion or the digestive tract	Dyspepsia, indigestion or stomach discomfort
-pnea (NEE-uh)	Breathing	Eupnea, normal breathing

SUFFIXES FOR PROFESSIONALS AND SPECIALTIES		
SUFFIX	MEANING	EXAMPLE
-thorax (THOR-ax)	Chest	Hemothorax, when blood collects between the chest wall and the lungs
-uria (you-REE-uh)	Relating to the urine	Hematuria, bloody urine

GRAMMATICAL SUFFIXES

Just like any other great language, medical terminology has its own grammatical conventions. Many suffixes are used purely for this purpose, indicating how a word functions. They often signal that a term "pertains to" the word's root.

It's important to remember that in medicine we try to avoid labeling patients by their diseases. Rather, we prefer to use person-first language. Rather than calling somebody a "hemophiliac" (a use of the -ac suffix), it is more polite, accurate, and patient-centric to say "a person with hemophilia."

Here's a look at important grammatical suffixes, and how they change the function of the words they're attached to.

GRAMMATICAL SUFFIXES		
SUFFIX	GRAMMATICAL FUNCTION	EXAMPLE
-ac (ACK)	Pertaining to; one afflicted with	Cardiac, heart
-al (ALL)	Pertaining to	Congenital, present from birth
-ar (ARR)	Pertaining to	Pustular, a skin rash filled with pus
-ary (AIRY)	Pertaining to	Biliary, relating to structures of the biliary tract

(continued)

(continued from previous page)

GRAMMATICAL SUFFIXES		
SUFFIX	GRAMMATICAL FUNCTION	EXAMPLE
-ation (AY-shunn)	A process	Endotracheal intubation, the procedure of placing and securing an artificial airway
-eal (EE-uhl)	Pertaining to	Esophageal, relating to the esophagus
-gen (JEN)	Substance or agent that generates an effect	Pathogen, a bacterium, virus, or other organism that causes disease
-ial (EE-all)	Of, relating to, connected	Facial, relating to the face
-ic (ICK)	Pertaining to	Hepatic, pertaining to the liver
-ine (IN)	Of, pertaining to	Medicine, the science of diagnosis, treatment, and prevention of disease
-ism (IZ-mm)	A condition or disease	Bruxism, a condition of teeth grinding
-ium (EE-um)	Structure, tissue	Myocardium, heart muscle tissue
-oid (OID)	Resembling, bearing resemblance to	Myxoid, a connective tissue tumor that resembles mucus
-osis (OH-sis)	A condition, disease, or process	Acidosis, a physiological process that makes a tissue or solution (often blood) more acidic
-ous (US)	Pertaining to	Cancerous, pertaining to cancer
-tic (TICK)	Pertaining to	Sclerotic, pertaining to hard, fibrous, or scar-like tissue
-ula (YOU-la), **-ule** (YOU'LL)	Small	Venule, very small vein

COMMON SUFFIXES IN MEDICAL TERMINOLOGY

Since not all suffixes fit into the above categories, we'll close out this chapter by looking at some commonly used suffixes we haven't studied yet. You'll find that this batch includes many suffixes describing position, direction, shape, color, and other physical characteristics.

OTHER COMMON SUFFIXES		
SUFFIX	MEANING	EXAMPLE
-ad (AD)	Toward, in the direction of	Cephalad, toward the head
-ase (ACE)	Enzyme	Lactase, the gut enzyme that digests the sugar lactose
-cyte (SITE)	Cell	Myocyte, a muscle cell
-cytosis (sy-TOH-sis)	An abundance of cells	Leukocytosis, an abnormally high amount of white blood cells
-drome (DROME)	Run, pace, timing	Prodrome, an early symptom or warning
-esis (EE-sis)	Pertaining to a condition, disease, or symptom	Diuresis, increased excretion of urine (either pathologic or due to medications)
-form (FORM)	Similar in appearance to, having the form of	Schizophreniform, a psychotic condition that resembles schizophrenia but only lasts one to six months
-genesis (JEN-eh-sis)	Creation of	Osteogenesis, bone formation
-geusia (GEEZ-ee-uh, rhymes with cheese)	Taste	Dysgeusia, foul taste, often metallic

(continued)

(continued from previous page)

OTHER COMMON SUFFIXES		
SUFFIX	MEANING	EXAMPLE
-gnosis (NO-sis)	Knowledge, identification of	Diagnosis, identification of the cause of an illness
-ion (EE-on)	A state or condition, an action or process	Ectropion, when the lower eyelid droops away from the eye
-mimetic (mim-EH-tick)	Similar to or resembling	Sympathomimetic, a substance or experience that produces a fight or flight response (triggering the sympathetic nervous system)
-morph (MORF)	Shape or form	Mesomorph, a muscular body type
-ol (ALL)	An alcohol	Ethanol, the type of alcohol in commercially available intoxicants
-ose (OSE)	Sugar	Lactose, the sugar naturally found in dairy products
-phil (FILL), **-philic** (FILL-ick)	Loving, attraction for	Lipophilic, the tendency to dissolve in or combine with fats
-physis (FYE-sis)	Growth	Epiphysis, the end of bones, containing the "growth plates"
-plasia (PLAY-zhuh)	Formation, development	Hyperplasia, enlargement of tissue due to creation of more cells
-plasm (PLA-zm)	Living substance, tissue	Protoplasm, the colorless material comprising the living part of a cell
-poeisis (po-EE-sis)	Production, generation	Hematopoiesis, production of blood cells

OTHER COMMON SUFFIXES		
SUFFIX	MEANING	EXAMPLE
-prandial (pran-DEE-uhl)	Eating, meals	Postprandial, the time immediately after eating a meal
-stalsis (STALL-sis)	Contraction	Peristalsis, the coordinated contraction of the smooth muscle of the digestive tract that propels food forward
-stasis (STAY-sis)	Stopped, standing, not moving	Hemostasis, to stop bleeding
-stenosis (sten-OH-sis)	Abnormal narrowing of a blood vessel or other tubular organ or structure	Restenosis, when an artery that was previously opened becomes narrowed again
-tension (TEN-shun), **-tensive** (TEN-sive)	Pressure	Normotension, normal blood pressure
-tion (SHUN)	A state or process	Lacrimation, the process of crying, tear production
-toxic (TOX-ick)	Poisonous, directly damaging	Hepatotoxic, a substance that directly injures the liver
-trophy (TROW-fee)	Nourishment, development	Hypertrophy, enlargement of tissue due to an increase in the size of cells
-y (EE)	Relating to a state, condition or process	Surgery, the process of performing an operation

KEY TAKEAWAYS

Congratulations! You have learned root words, prefixes, and now suffixes. With that accomplished, you now have mastery of the building blocks for thousands of medical terms. That is a big achievement, and you should be proud of yourself!

By the way, remember "esophagogastroduodenoscopy" (EGD) from the beginning of this chapter? You may have figured out its meaning: a procedure (-scopy) for viewing the upper digestive tract, the esophagus (eso-), stomach (gastro-), and duodenum (duodeno-).

In this chapter, we learned suffixes related to surgeries, procedures, diseases, grammar, and many other commonly used terms. Here are the key takeaways from this chapter:

- Many suffixes indicate that a term describes physical characteristics (for example, color, shape, or function).

- There are suffixes that signal a word describes procedures and surgeries.

- Many suffixes indicate a condition or pathology.

- Suffixes are used as grammatical tools to complete a medical term, denoting how the term functions.

QUIZ

1. Your doctor plans to perform an arthrocentesis. What does the procedure do to your joint?

   a. fuses the joint

   b. breaks the bones

   c. removes joint fluid

2. If your doctor tells you that you have "hepatomegaly," they are saying that your liver is____.

   a. ruptured

   b. hardened

   c. enlarged

3. Polyuria means an excessive amount of ____.

   a. urine

   b. blood

   c. gas

4. What does the suffix "-oid" mean?

   a. old

   b. resembling

   c. small

5. "Hydrophilic" literally means _____ water.

   a. afraid of

   b. opposite of

   c. loving

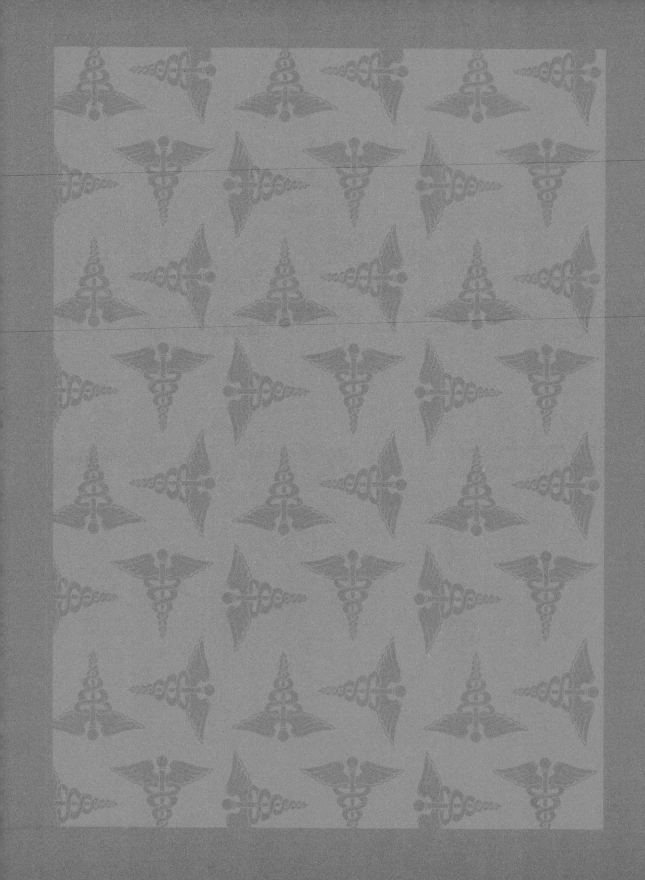

CHAPTER 7

HOMOPHONES, EPONYMS, ACRONYMS, ABBREVIATIONS, AND SYMBOLS

You now have the tools to create and understand nearly every medical term that is built from a prefix, root, and suffix. You're extremely well-equipped to make sense of whatever medical language you encounter, but there are some final challenges ahead.

Some medical terms are homophones, words that are pronounced the same but have different meanings. It is important that you are aware of these so you can avoid mistaking one for the other.

The medical language also includes innumerable eponyms, which are diseases, procedures, and other terms named after people. As such, they are not built from the prefixes, roots, and suffixes you have studied.

Medicine is filled with commonly used acronyms and abbreviations. Before the electronic medical record, documenting everything by hand was tedious, so acronyms reducing long words or phrases to key letters ("electroencephalogram" to "EEG") and other abbreviations became commonplace. Many of those have survived the digital transformation and are still commonly used in medical practice.

Finally, you will want to become familiar with important symbols used in medicine, many of which you've already seen in other contexts.

So, to make your understanding of medical terms complete, we'll spend this final chapter learning and recognizing the tricky medical lexical situations that don't fit the usual patterns. Don't worry. You're more than up for the task.

HOMOPHONES AND SOUND-ALIKES

Homophones are words that are pronounced the same way but have different meanings. For example, consider the terms "aural" (related to the ear) and "oral" (by mouth). Imagine giving a medication by mouth that was actually supposed to be put in the ear, or vice versa. That certainly would not be ideal. Along with homophones, you'll encounter medical terms that are pronounced differently but sound enough alike that they could be mistaken for each other when spoken aloud. This table presents of the most easily confused sound-alike medical terms so you can be alert for errors when you hear them. Some people find it helpful to speak each word out loud to help remember which is which.

SOUND-ALIKE MEDICAL TERMS			
WORD AND MEANING	PRONUNCIATION	WORD AND MEANING	PRONUNCIATION
Abduction: moving away from the sagittal plane From the same root word as "to abduct" or take away from	ab-DUCK-shun	**Adduction:** moving toward a position or the midline	add-DUCK-shun
Aberrant: deviating from normal	uh-BEAR-ant	**Apparent:** obvious, visible, evident	app-AIR-ent
Access: to approach or enter, often in terms of "venous access"	ACK-sess	**Axis:** an imaginary line about which an object rotates Often refers to the spinal column	AX-iss
Agonist: a substance that causes a physiological response when binding to a receptor	AG-on-ist	**Antagonist:** a substance that interferes with the binding of an agonist	ant-AG-on-ist
Anuresis: lack of urine production	AN-yurr-EE-sis	**Enuresis:** involuntary urination, often at night	ENN-yurr-EE-sis
Apophysis: a bony protuberance	ap-PAH-fih-sis	**Epiphysis:** the end portion of a long bone or "shaft"	epp-IFF-ih-sis
Apposition: setting one object next to another	APP-uh-ZIH-shun	**Opposition:** in contrast, antithesis, against	OPP-oh-ZIH-shun
Aural: pertaining to the ear	AW-rall	**Oral:** pertaining to the mouth	OR-all

(continued)

(continued from previous page)

SOUND-ALIKE MEDICAL TERMS			
WORD AND MEANING	PRONUNCIATION	WORD AND MEANING	PRONUNCIATION
Calculus: an aggregation of minerals, bone, or a "stone" (e.g., kidney stone or gallstone)	CAL-cue-luss	**Calcaneus:** heel bone	cal-CANE-ee-us
*Cor: pertaining to the heart (e.g., Coronary artery)	CORE	***Core:** the central part of something	CORE
Creatine: a nitrogen-based molecule found in muscles, brain, and blood	CREE-uh-teen	**Creatinine:** a substance, commonly measured in blood to assess kidney function	cree-AT-ih-neen
*Dermatome: an area of skin supplied by nerves from a single spinal root	DER-muh-tome	***Dermatome:** a surgical instrument to produce thin slices of skin for use in skin grafts	DER-muh-tome
Diaphysis: the shaft of a long bone	dye-A-fih-sis	**Diastasis:** a predisposition to a certain disease	dye-A-stuh-sis
Dysphagia: difficulty eating	dis-FAY-juh	**Dysphasia:** difficulty speaking	dis-FAY-zhuh
Galactorrhea: abnormal flow of breast milk	guh-LACK-torr-EE-uh	**Galacturia:** urine that resembles milk	guh-lackt-YURR-EE-uh
Humeral: pertaining to the humerus (arm) bone	HYOO-mer-uhl	**Humoral:** pertaining to a body fluid	hu-MOR-uhl
Hypophysis: a "stalk," often referring to the pituitary gland	hi-PAH-fiss-iss	**Hypothesis:** a proposed explanation of a phenomenon	hi-PAH-this-iss

SOUND-ALIKE MEDICAL TERMS			
WORD AND MEANING	PRONUNCIATION	WORD AND MEANING	PRONUNCIATION
*Ileum: the last portion of the small intestine	ILL-ee-um	*Ilium: the superior portion of the pelvis	ILL-ee-um
*Lice: tiny biting insects	LICE	*Lyse: breaking down, often of a cell or cell components	LICE
Malleolus: a bony projection of the ankle	muh-LAY-oh-luss	Malleus: a tiny bone of the inner ear	MAL-ee-us
Melanotic: having black pigmentation (melanin)	meh-lan-OTT-ick	Melenic: black tarry stool	meh-LEN-ick
Metacarpal: the long bones of the hand	met-uh-CARP-uhl	Metatarsal: the long bones of the foot	met-uh-TARS-uhl
Metaphysis: the wide portion at the end of a long bone	met-A-fiss-is	Metastasis: spread of disease, often via the bloodstream or lymphatics	met-A-stuh-sis
*Osteal: relating to bone	OSS-tee-uhl	*Ostial: an opening (os)	OSS-tee-uhl
Palpation: to examine by touch	pal-PAY-shun	Palpitation: the sensation of the heart beating, often irregularly	pal-pih-TAY-shun
Peroneal: relating to the fibula or outer side of the leg	per-OH-nee-uhl	Perineal: relating to the perineum, the area between the anus and the vulva or scrotum	per-ih-NEE-uhl
*Plural: more than one	PLURR-uhl	*Pleural: the space between the lungs/heart and chest wall	PLURR-uhl

(continued)

(continued from previous page)

SOUND-ALIKE MEDICAL TERMS			
WORD AND MEANING	PRONUNCIATION	WORD AND MEANING	PRONUNCIATION
Profuse: lavish, bountiful	pro-FUZE	**Perfuse:** to flow, flow through, or spread	per-FUZE
Prostate: the prostate gland	PROH-state	**Prostrate:** lying prone	PROH-strait
Tract: a passageway of tissue	TRACKT	**Track:** a pathway	TRACK
*Vesicle: a small blister or fluid-filled sac	VES-ick-uhl	***Vesical:** relating to the urinary bladder	VES-ick-uhl
*Viscus: an internal organ	VISS-cuss	***Viscous:** a thick or dense substance	VISS-cuss

* indicates word pairs which are pronounced identically (homophones).

EPONYMS

Many medical terms are eponyms, named for people who discovered diseases, pioneered new surgeries, or first described physiological phenomena. Some eponyms are named after characters in mythology or literature, or even famous people. In recent years, there has been a major effort to stop using eponyms and instead use standard medical terminology. Nevertheless, many eponyms are still in use, so let's take a look at the ones you're most likely to encounter. You might see some of these with or without a possessive, such as Hodgkin's lymphoma or Hodgkin lymphoma.

EPONYMS		
MEDICAL TERM	NAMED AFTER	DEFINITION
Achilles tendon	Achilles, Greek mythological character	The tendon that connects the calf muscle to the heel
Addison's disease	Thomas Addison, English physician and scientist	A disease that leads to adrenal insufficiency

EPONYMS		
MEDICAL TERM	NAMED AFTER	DEFINITION
Alzheimer's disease	Alois Alzheimer, German psychiatrist	A common form of dementia
Apgar score	Virginia Apgar, American obstetrician	A quick assessment of the health of a newborn baby
Bell's palsy	Charles Bell, Scottish surgeon	A type of facial paralysis
Crohn's disease	Burrill Bernard Crohn, American gastroenterologist	A type of inflammatory bowel disease
Cushing syndrome	Harvey Cushing, American neurosurgeon	Conditions leading to excessive cortisol
Down's syndrome	John Langdon Down, British physician	A genetic disorder caused by inheriting three (rather than two) copies of chromosome 21
Epley's maneuver	John Epley, American physician	An exercise to treat symptoms of benign paroxysmal positional vertigo
Eustachian tube	Bartolomeo Eustachi, Italian anatomist	The small passageway that connects the throat to the inner ear
Fallopian tube	Gabriele Falloppio, Italian anatomist	The conduits between the ovaries and uterus
Foley catheter	Frederic Eugene Basil Foley, American urologist	An indwelling urinary catheter
Fowler's position	George Ryerson Fowler, American surgeon	A patient on their back in a semi-seated position, with their upper body elevated
Frank's sign	Sanders T. Frank, American pulmonologist	A diagonal earlobe crease associated with cardiovascular disease

(continued)

(continued from previous page)

EPONYMS		
MEDICAL TERM	NAMED AFTER	DEFINITION
Graves' disease	Robert James Graves, Irish surgeon	The most common cause of hyperthyroidism
Heimlich maneuver	Henry Heimlich, American thoracic surgeon	Abdominal thrusts to stop choking
Hodgkin's lymphoma	Thomas Hodgkin, British physician	A type of lymphatic system cancer
Lou Gehrig's disease	Lou Gehrig, American baseball player who had this condition	Amyotrophic Lateral Sclerosis (ALS), a progressive, degenerative neurological condition
Mohs surgery	Frederic E. Mohs, American general surgeon	The removal of skin cancer by microscopic layers
Parkinson's disease	James Parkinson, English surgeon	A degenerative disorder of the central nervous system
Tommy John surgery	Tommy John, the first major league pitcher to undergo the surgery	Ulnar collateral ligament reconstructive surgery

ACRONYMS

Now we arrive at another, slightly controversial, set of medical terms. As I mentioned, abbreviations make our documentation and communication faster. Many, if not most, abbreviations in medical terminology are acronyms: terms formed using key letters of a word or series of words. However, the usefulness of acronyms comes at the cost of potential confusion, particularly for people who aren't familiar with them or who are outside of the health-care profession. Health-care providers should make every effort to limit acronyms, but you're still likely to encounter them. So, familiarize yourself with these key examples, many of which relate to disease states.

Most of these acronyms are pronounced by spelling out the letters, such as "A-K-I" or "C-A-D." However, some are pronounced as words, such as AIDS.

ACRONYMS	
ACRONYM	MEANING
AAA ("triple A")	Abdominal Aortic Aneurysm
AF, AFib	Atrial Fibrillation
AFL	Atrial Flutter
AIDS*	Acquired Immunodeficiency Syndrome
AKI	Acute Kidney Injury
ALF	Acute Liver Failure
ARDS*	Acute (or Adult) Respiratory Distress Syndrome
AS	Aortic Stenosis
BPBPR	Bright Red Blood Per Rectum
BPH	Benign Prostatic Hyperplasia
CAD	Coronary Artery Disease
CHF	Congestive Heart Failure
CKD	Chronic Kidney Disease
COPD	Chronic Obstructive Pulmonary Disease
CVA	Cerebral Vascular Attack (a stroke)
DKA	Diabetic Ketoacidosis
DM1	Diabetes Mellitus Type 1
DM2	Diabetes Mellitus Type 2
DVT	Deep Vein Thrombosis
ESRD	End-Stage Renal Disease
FB	Foreign Body
GERD*	Gastroesophageal Reflux Disease
HIV	Human Immunodeficiency Virus
HLD	Hyperlipidemia

(continued)

(*continued from previous page*)

ACRONYMS	
ACRONYM	MEANING
HTN	Hypertension
IBD	Inflammatory Bowel Disease
IBS	Irritable Bowel Syndrome
LBO	Large Bowel Obstruction
MI	Myocardial Infarction (heart attack)
MS	Multiple Sclerosis
MVA	Motor Vehicle Accident
N/V	Nausea and Vomiting
OSA	Obstructive Sleep Apnea
PAD, PVD	Peripheral Arterial Disease, Peripheral Vascular Disease
PE	Pulmonary Embolism
PEA	Pulseless Electrical Activity (a form of cardiac arrest)
PID	Pelvic Inflammatory Disease
PNA	Pneumonia
SBO	Small Bowel Obstruction
UGIB, LGIB	Upper (or Lower) Gastrointestinal Bleed
UTI	Urinary Tract Infection
VF	Ventricular Fibrillation (a form of cardiac arrest)
VT	Ventricular Tachycardia

* indicates the term should be pronounced as a word, rather than spelled out.

PHARMACEUTICAL ABBREVIATIONS

The pharmacy has its own set of acronyms that are commonly used. Many come from Latin terms, which can be quite confusing when you first see them. It took me a while to understand why an intravenous infusion was shorthanded as "gtt." That's short for the Latin "guttae," or "drops," so "gtt" indicates medication slowly dripped into a patient's bloodstream. You will find many of these terms in medication dosing and instructions.

PHARMACEUTICAL ABBREVIATIONS	
ABBREVIATION	MEANING
AC	Ante Cibum (before meals)
ABx	Antibiotics
ART	Antiretroviral Therapy
ASAP*	As Soon As Possible
BID	Bis In Die (twice daily)
Cap	Capsule
D/C	Discontinued
Gtt	Guttae (drip or infusion)
HAART*	Highly Active Antiretroviral Therapy
IM	Intramuscular
IV	Intravenous
IVP	Intravenous Push
K	Potassium (from the Latin word "kalium")
mEq	Milliequivalents
mg	Milligrams
mL	Milliliters
Na	Sodium (from the Latin word "natrium")

(continued)

(continued from previous page)

| PHARMACEUTICAL ABBREVIATIONS ||
ABBREVIATION	MEANING
NS	Normal Saline (0.9% sodium chloride)
PC	Post Cibum (after meals)
PR	Per Rectum
PO	Per Os (by mouth)
PRN	Pro Re Nata (as needed)
QD	Quaque Die (every day)
QID	Quater In Die (four times daily)
Q2h, Q3h, Q4h	Every two, three, or four hours
QAM	Every Morning
QHS	Quaque Hora Somni (every night at bedtime)
QPM	Every Evening
SC or SubQ	Subcutaneous
STAT*	Statium (immediately)
TID	Ter In Die (three times daily)
TPN	Total Parenteral Nutrition
Tab	Tablet

* indicates the term should be pronounced as a word, rather than spelled out.

SURGICAL AND TREATMENT ABBREVIATIONS

Up next, we have important abbreviations that relate to surgeries and other procedures. You'll find these commonly used terms in patient notes, operative reports, and charts.

SURGICAL AND TREATMENT ABBREVIATIONS	
ABBREVIATION	MEANING
AKA, BKA	Above the Knee Amputation, Below the Knee Amputation
BLS	Basic Life Saving
BMT	Bone Marrow Transplant
BSO	Bilateral Salpingectomy Oophorectomy
CABG*	Coronary Artery Bypass Graft
CPR	Cardiopulmonary Resuscitation
DC	Discharged (from the hospital or clinic); Discontinue (often in regard to an order)
EBL	Estimated Blood Loss
ECT	Electroconvulsive Therapy
ET	Endotracheal Tube
HD	Hemodialysis
HRT	Hormone Replacement Therapy
ICU	Intensive Care Unit
IUD	Intrauterine Device
IVF	IV Fluids; In Vitro Fertilization
KVO	Keep Vein Open
LP	Lumbar Puncture
NG	Nasogastric (tube)
NSAID*	Non-Steroidal Anti-Inflammatory Drug

(continued)

(continued from previous page)

SURGICAL AND TREATMENT ABBREVIATIONS	
ABBREVIATION	MEANING
PEG*	Percutaneous Gastrostomy Tube
PPI	Proton Pump Inhibitor
PT	Physical Therapy
RRT	Rapid Response Team
RT	Respiratory Therapy
TAH	Total Abdominal Hysterectomy
TAVR*	Transcatheter Aortic Valve Replacement
THA	Total Hip Arthroplasty (Hip Replacement)
TKA	Total Knee Arthroplasty (Knee Replacement)

* indicates the term should be pronounced as a word, rather than spelled out.

ABBREVIATIONS USED IN ASSESSMENT, DIAGNOSTICS, AND DOCUMENTATION

I have one final list of acronyms for you. If you're going to be using medical terminology, chances are high that you'll come across many of these abbreviations relating to diagnostic tools, tests, and other key aspects of medical practice. In fact, I use quite a few of these on a daily basis.

DIAGNOSTICS AND DOCUMENTATION ABBREVIATIONS	
ABBREVIATION	MEANING
A1c or HbA1c	Glycated Hemoglobin (a blood test)
ABG	Arterial blood gas
Ad Lib	Ad Libitum (Move freely)
BS, BG	Blood Sugar or Blood Glucose
BCx	Blood Cultures

DIAGNOSTICS AND DOCUMENTATION ABBREVIATIONS	
ABBREVIATION	MEANING
BM	Bowel Movement
BMP	Basic Metabolic Panel (a blood test)
BSA	Body Surface Area
Bx	Biopsy
CBC	Comprehensive Blood Count (a blood test)
CMP	Comprehensive Metabolic Panel (a blood test)
CN	Cranial Nerve
CNS	Central Nervous System
CO2	Carbon Dioxide
CSF	Cerebrospinal Fluid
CT or CAT Scan	Computed Tomography Scan
CXR	Chest X Ray
DBP	Diastolic Blood Pressure
DPOA	Designated Power of Attorney
Dx	Diagnosis
ECG, EKG	Electrocardiogram (K is from the German spelling)
ED, ER	Emergency Department, Emergency Room
EEG	Electroencephalogram
EGD	Esophagogastroduodenoscopy
EMS	Emergency Medical Services
EtOH	Ethanol (or alcohol)
ETT	Exercise Treadmill Test
Fx	Fracture; Function
Hgb or Hb	Hemoglobin

(continued)

(continued from previous page)

DIAGNOSTICS AND DOCUMENTATION ABBREVIATIONS	
ABBREVIATION	MEANING
HR	Heart Rate
LFTs	Liver Function Tests
MAP*	Mean Arterial Pressure
MRI	Magnetic Resonance Imaging
NPO	Nil Per Os (nothing by mouth)
OD	Oculus Dexter (right eye)
OS	Oculus Sinister (left eye)
OU	Oculus Uterque (both eyes)
PLT	Platelets
RA	Room Air
RBC	Red Blood Cells
ROM*	Range Of Motion
SBP	Systolic Blood Pressure
SNF	Skilled Nursing Facility
SOB	Shortness Of Breath
T	Temperature
UA	Urinalysis
VBG	Venous Blood Gas
w/ or c/	With
w/o or s/	Without
WBC	White Blood Cells
YO	Years Old

* indicates the term should be pronounced as a word, rather than spelled out.

SYMBOLS

You have made it to the final table in this book, and that's no small feat. Since you have put in so much work, it seems fitting to end with a relatively easy list; in fact, you won't even have to memorize any words. This table shares some important symbols commonly used in health care. Since many are in general use, you'll find quite a few familiar icons here.

SYMBOLS	
SYMBOL	MEANING
≈	Approximately
@	At
Δ	Change
°	Degree
↓	Down or low
=	Equal to
♂	Female
>	Greater than
<	Less than
♀	Male
μ	Micro
-	Minus or negative
+	Plus or positive
↑	Up or high

A FINAL NOTE

Congratulations for making it all the way through this book! We've covered a tremendous amount of material, and you should be proud of yourself.

This is likely just the beginning of your journey with medical terminology. Whether you are starting your medical training, are already a seasoned practitioner, or are a patient or caregiver, there will always be more to learn and master. But I hope working your way through these pages has taught you how to confidently break down and understand whatever new terms come your way. Keep this book handy so you can refer to it if you need to research new words. Most of all, I hope the time you put into studying medical terminology improves your communication and connection with the medical field, whatever your situation. We are all better off when we are more connected.

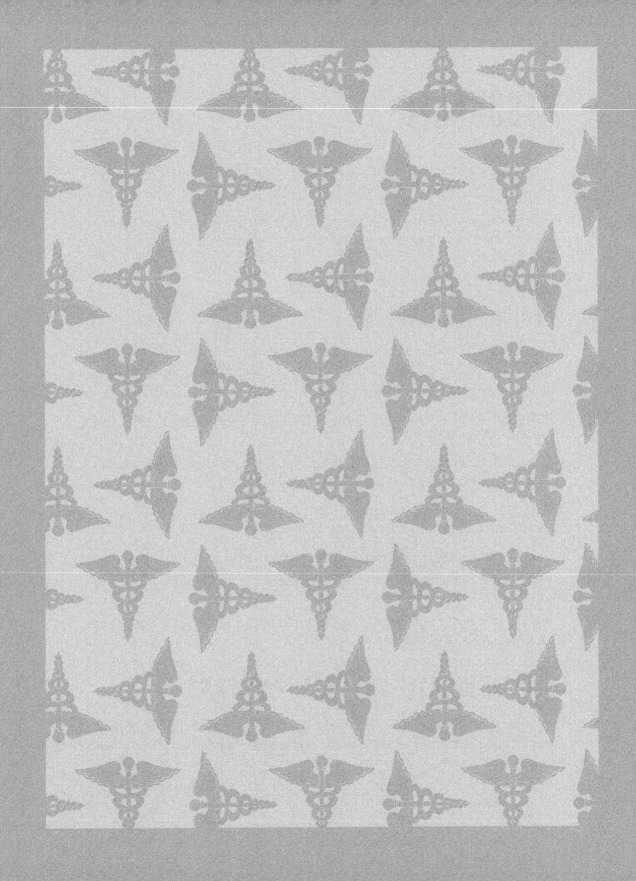

RESOURCES

Here's a collection of resources that will help enhance your study of medicine and medical terminology, including some of my favorite sources and tools.

BOOKS FOR FURTHER STUDY OF MEDICAL TERMINOLOGY

Learn Medical Terminology: Flash Card Activities, Instructional Videos, & Complete Guide to Master Medical Terms for Healthcare Professionals. Helpful Matthew, et al. 2020.

Medical Terminology: A Living Language, 6th ed. Bonnie F. Fremgen and Suzanne S. Frucht. 2015.

Medical Terminology: An Easy and Practical Guide to Better Understand, Pronounce, and Memorize Terms. Nathan Orwell. 2021.

Medical Terminology: Learn to Pronounce, Understand and Memorize Over 2000 Medical Terms (Audiobook). Matt Clark. 2019.

Medical Terminology: The Best and Most Effective Way to Memorize, Pronounce and Understand Medical Terms, 2nd ed. M. Mastenbjörk MD, S. Meloni MD, D. Andersson. 2015.

Medical Terminology for Dummies, 3rd ed. Beverley Henderson CMT-R HRT, Jennifer L. Dorsey PhD, et al. 2020.

MEDICAL COURSES AND STUDY PROGRAMS

Amboss. This is a comprehensive study and reference app for medical trainees and clinicians. It is recommended for experienced health-care trainees. amboss.com

Boards & Beyond. This is an online study resource for medical students, primarily for board preparation. boardsbeyond.com

Geeky Medics. This is a comprehensive study resource focused on clinical skills, procedures, and medical studies in general. geekymedics.com

Online MedEd. This is by far one of the best medical study resources available taught via short, high-yield educational videos. onlinemeded.org

Osmosis by Elsevier. This is a wonderful resource for easy-to-understand medical education for medical trainees and the general public. osmosis.org

Nursecepts. This is a resource for student nurses. nursecepts.com

Sketchy. A novel and popular study resource for all things medical, Sketchy uses images to help with memorizations and is a favorite among medical and nursing students. sketchy.com

Teach Me Anatomy. This app is great for health-care professionals and medical students. It contains high-yield articles, images, diagrams, and quizzes. teachmeanatomy.info

PODCASTS

Curbsiders Podcast. This is one of my favorite education and entertainment medical podcasts. thecurbsiders.com

Curious Clinicians Podcast. "The medical podcast that asks why" dives deep into medical mysteries that are always informative and entertaining. curiousclinicians.com

YOUTUBE CHANNELS

Alila Medical Media. This channel presents simple and clear mini lectures on medical topics.

Armando Hasudungan. This channel offers detailed and informative medical diagrams that are very informative for medical studies.

Dr. Najeeb Lectures. These lectures dive deep into physiology and pathology for clinicians.

Harvard Medical School. These high-quality medical videos are for health profession students and the general population.

Healthcare Triage. This is a comprehensive resource for healthcare topics and current events.

Khan Academy Medicine. This is one of the best online education platforms available and has great medical education lectures.

Nucleus Medical Media. This channel provides great, brief medical education videos and animations.

One Minute Medical School. This channel provides short videos that cover a wide array of diseases and conditions.

Strong Medicine. This channel provides useful videos for medical trainees and professionals.

Zero to Finals. This channel provides wonderful medical diagrams and instructional lectures.

REFERENCES

American Institute of Medical Sciences & Education. "All Essential Medical Terms in One Place." *AIMS Education*, American Institute of Medical Sciences & Education. aimseducation.edu/blog/all-essential -medical-terms.

Corriero, Claudia. "The Anatomy of Medical Jargon (Part 2)." Pocket Anatomy. pocketanatomy.com/teaching-anatomy/the-anatomy-of -medical-jargon.

Des Moines University Medical & Health Sciences. "Basics." February 4, 2011. dmu.edu/medterms/basics.

EnglishClub. "Medical English Vocabulary." 2022. englishclub.com /english-for-work/medical-vocabulary.htm.

English Hints. "30+ Medical Prefixes and Roots Worth Learning." 2022. englishhints.com/medical-prefixes.html.

Global RPh. "The Clinician's Ultimate Reference." 2021. globalrph.com.

Meditec. "Sound Alike Words." meditec.com/resourcestools/medical-words /sound-alike-words.

Nursecepts. "Student Nurse Resource." 2017. nursecepts.com.

Online Etymology Dictionary. 2022. etymonline.com.

Repas, Laszlo. *Basics of Medical Terminology: Latin and Greek Origins: Textbook for First Year Medical Students*. 2013. medi-lingua.hu/home.

St. George's University. "75 Must-Know Medical Terms, Abbreviations, and Acronyms." 2022. https://www.sgu.edu/blog/medical/medical-terms -abbreviations-and-acronyms.

Wulff, Henrik R. "The Language of Medicine." *Journal of the Royal Society of Medicine* 97, no. 4 (March 31, 2004): 187–88. doi.org/10.1258/jrsm .97.4.187.

INDEX

A

A1c (glycated hemoglobin), 130
AAA (abdominal aortic
    aneurysm), 125
A/an- prefix, 87
Ab/abs- prefix, 80, 92
Abbreviations
  diagnostic, 130–132
  pharmaceutical, 127–128
  surgical and treatment, 129–130
  use of, 118
Abdomen
  cavity, 24, 32
  defined, 25
  quadrants, 24, 28
  regions, 24, 29–30
Abdominal cavity, 32
Abduction, vs. adduction, 119
Aberrant, vs. apparent, 119
ABG (arterial blood gas), 130
ABx (antibiotics), 127
AC (ante cibum), 127
Acanth- prefix, 87
Access, vs. axis, 119
Achilles tendon, 122
Acou- root, 70
Acronyms, 118, 124–126
Acr/o- root, 66
-ac suffix, 109
-acusis suffix, 107
Addison's disease, 122

Adduction, vs. abduction, 119
Aden/o- root, 46
Adip/o- root, 47
Ad Lib (ad libitum), 130
Ad- prefix, 80, 92
Adren/o- root, 46
-ad suffix, 111
Aer/o- root, 70
Aesthesi- root, 52
AF/AFib (atrial fibrillation), 125
AFL (atrial flutter), 125
Agonist, vs. antagonist, 119
AIDS (acquired immunodeficiency
    syndrome), 125
AKA (above the knee
    amputation), 129
AKI (acute kidney injury), 125
Albin/o- prefix, 86
Alb/o- prefix, 86
ALF (acute liver failure), 125
Alge/algesia root, 52, 70
Algi/o- root, 70
All/o- prefix, 87
Allo- prefix, 92
-al suffix, 109
Alveol/o- root, 42
Alzheimer's disease, 123
Ambi- prefix, 87
Amni/o- root, 58
Ana- prefix, 81
Anatomical planes, 20–21

Anatomic position, 21
Andr/o- prefix, 92
Andr/o- root, 60
Angi/o- root, 40
Aniso- prefix, 87
Ankyl/o- root, 49
Antagonist, vs. agonist, 119
Antebrachial region, 26
Antecubital region, 26
Ante- prefix, 81
Anterior body regions, 25–26
Anterior direction, 22, 73
Anter/o- prefix, 92
Anti- prefix, 87
Antonyms, 92–93
Anuresis, vs. enuresis, 119
Aort/o- root, 40
Apgar score, 123
Apophysis, vs. epiphysis, 119
Ap/o- prefix, 81
Apo- prefix, 87
Apparent, vs. aberrant, 119
Append/o- root, 44
Apposition, vs. opposition, 119
ARDS (acute/adult respiratory
    distress syndrome), 125
-ar suffix, 109
ART (antiretroviral therapy), 127
Arthr/o- root, 49
Articul- root, 49
-ary suffix, 109
AS (aortic stenosis), 125
ASAP (as soon as possible), 127
-ase suffix, 111
-asthenia suffix, 103
Atel/o- root, 42
Ather/o- root, 40
-ation suffix, 110

-atresia suffix, 103
Atri/o- root, 40
Audi/o- root, 54
Aural, vs. oral, 119
Auricul/o- root, 54
Auto- prefix, 87, 92
Axial plane, 20
Axillary region, 26
Axill/o- root, 66
Axis, vs. access, 119
Azo/to- root, 56

B

Bacter/i- root, 70
Balan/o- root, 60
BCx (blood cultures), 130
Bell's palsy, 123
BG (blood glucose), 130
BID (bis in die), 127
-bilia suffix, 103
Bio- prefix, 92
Bi- prefix, 84
BKA (below the knee
    amputation), 129
Blast- root, 70
Blephar/o- root, 54, 66
BLS (basic life saving), 129
BM (bowel movement), 131
BMP (basic metabolic panel), 131
BMT (bone marrow transplant), 129
Body
  anatomical planes, 20–21
  cavities, 24, 32
  directions, 22–23, 73–75
  organization of, 33
  positions, 21–22
  quiz, 34
  regions, 24–31

Bovine- prefix, 88
BPBPR (bright red blood
　　per rectum), 125
BPH (benign prostatic
　　hyperplasia), 125
Brachial region, 26
Brachi/o- root, 66
Brachy- prefix, 88
Brady- prefix, 88, 92
Bronch/i/io- root, 42
Bronchiol/i- root, 42
BS (blood sugar), 130
BSA (body surface area), 131
BSO (bilateral salpingectomy
　　oophorectomy), 129
Bucc/o- root, 66
Burs/o- root, 49
Bx (biopsy), 131

C

c/ (with), 132
CABG (coronary artery
　　bypass graft), 129
Caceneus, vs. calculus, 120
CAD (coronary artery disease), 125
Calcaneal region, 27
Calculus, vs. calceneus, 120
Canth/o- root, 66
Cap (capsule), 127
Capit/o- root, 66
-capnia suffix, 107
Capn/o- root, 42
-carcinoma suffix, 103
Carcin/o- root, 70
-cardia suffix, 108
Cardi/o- root, 41
Cardiovascular system, 40–41

Carpal region, 26
Carp/o- root, 49, 66
Cata- prefix, 88
CAT scan (computed tomography
　　scan), 131
Caudal direction, 22, 73
Caud/o- root, 66
Cavities, body, 24
CBC (comprehensive blood
　　count), 131
Cec/o- root, 44
-cele suffix, 103
Cellul/o- root, 70
-centesis suffix, 100
Centi- prefix, 85
Cephalic region, 25
Cephal/o- prefix, 94
Cephal/o- root, 52, 66
Ce pronunciation, 10
Cerebell/o- root, 52
Cerebr/o- root, 52
Cervical region, 24, 31
Cervic/o- root, 58, 66
Cheil/o- root, 47, 67
Chem/o- prefix, 88
CHF (congestive heart failure), 125
Chlor/o- prefix, 86
Cholecyst/o- root, 70
Chol/e- root, 44
Chondr/o- root, 49
Cho pronunciation, 10
-cidal suffix, 103
Cili/o- root, 70
Circum- prefix, 81
Cirrh/o- prefix, 87
Cis- prefix, 88, 92
CKD (chronic kidney disease), 125

-clasis suffix, 100
-clast suffix, 103
-clysis suffix, 101
CMP (comprehensive metabolic panel), 131
CN (cranial nerve), 131
CNS (central nervous system), 131
CO2 (carbon dioxide), 131
-coccus suffix, 103
Coccygeal region, 27, 31
Coccyx region, 24
Cochle/o- root, 54
Co/con/com- prefix, 88
Colon/o- root, 44
Col/o- root, 44
Color prefixes, 86–87
Colp/o- prefix, 94
Colp/o- root, 58
Conjunctiv/o- root, 54
Contra- prefix, 88
COPD (chronic obstructive pulmonary disease), 125
Cor, vs. core, 120
Core, vs. cor, 120
Corne/o- root, 54
Coronal plane, 21
Cortic/o- root, 70
Costal region, 26
Cost/o- root, 49, 70
CPR (cardiopulmonary resuscitation), 129
Cranial cavity, 32
Cranial direction, 22, 73
Cranial region, 25
Crani/o- prefix, 94
Crani/o- root, 52
Creatine, vs. creatinine, 120

Creatinine, vs. creatine, 120
-crine suffix, 108
-crit suffix, 101
Crohn's disease, 123
Crural region, 25
Cry/o- root, 71
Crypto- prefix, 88
Crypt/o- root, 71
CSF (cerebrospinal fluid), 131
CT (computed tomography scan), 131
Cu pronunciation, 10
Cushing syndrome, 123
Cutane/o- root, 47
Cutibal region, 27
CVA (cerebral vascular attack), 125
CXR (chest X ray), 131
Cyan/o- prefix, 86
Cyst/o- root, 56
-cyte suffix, 111
Cyt/o- root, 71
-cytosis suffix, 111

D

Dacry/o- root, 55
-dactyly suffix, 104
DBP (diastolic blood pressure), 131
DC (discharged/discontinue), 129
D/C (discontinued), 127
Deci- prefix, 85
Deep direction, 22, 74
Deka- prefix, 85
Deltoid region, 26
Dent/o- prefix, 94
Dent/o- root, 44
De- prefix, 88
Dermatome, 120
Dermat/o- root, 47

Derm/o- root, 47
-desis suffix, 101
Dextr/o- prefix, 81
Diagnostics
  abbreviations, 130–132
  suffixes, 100–102
Diaphragm, 24
Diaphysis, vs. diastasis, 120
Dia- prefix, 81
Diastasis, vs. diaphysis, 120
Diastol/e- root, 41
Digestive system, 44–45
Di- prefix, 81, 84
-dipsia suffix, 104
Directional root words, 73–75
Directions, body, 22–23
  prefixes, 80–83
  root words, 73–75
Dis- prefix, 88
Distal direction, 22, 74
DKA (diabetic ketoacidosis), 125
DM1 (diabetes mellitus type 1), 125
DM2 (diabetes mellitus type 2), 125
Dorsal cavity, 32
Dorsal direction, 23, 74
Dorsal recumbent position, 21
Dorsal region, 27
Down's syndrome, 123
DPOA (designated power of
    attorney), 131
-drome suffix, 111
Duoden/o- root, 44
DVT (deep vein thrombosis), 125
Dx (diagnosis), 131
-dynia suffix, 104
Dysphagia, vs. dysphasia, 120
Dysphasia, vs. dysphagia, 120
Dys- prefix, 88, 92, 94

E

-eal suffix, 110
EBL (estimated blood loss), 129
ECG (electrocardiogram), 131
Ec- prefix, 81
ECT (electroconvulsive therapy), 129
-ectasia suffix, 104
-ectomy suffix, 101
Ecto- prefix, 81
ED (emergency department), 131
-edema suffix, 104
EEG (electroencephalogram), 131
EGD (esophagogastroduodenos-
    copy), 131
EKG (electrocardiogram), 131
-emesis suffix, 104
-emia suffix, 104
EMS (emergency medical
    services), 131
Encephal/o- root, 52
Endocrine system, 46–47
Endocrin/o- root, 46
Endometri/o- root, 58
Endo- prefix, 92
En/endo- prefix, 81
Enter/o- root, 44, 71
Enuresis, vs. anuresis, 119
Eosin/o- prefix, 86
Epididym/o- root, 60
Epigastric region, 30
Epiphysis, vs. apophysis, 119
Epi- prefix, 82
Episi/o- root, 58, 71
Epley's maneuver, 123
Eponyms, 117–118, 122–124
ER (emergency room), 131
-er suffix, 108

Erythr/o- prefix, 86
-esis suffix, 111
Esophag/o- root, 44
ESRD (end-stage renal disease), 125
ET (endotracheal tube), 129
EtOH (ethanol), 131
ETT (exercise treadmill test), 131
Eu- prefix, 92
Eustachian tube, 123
Ex/extra- prefix, 82
Exo- prefix, 82, 92
External direction, 23, 74

F

Facial region, 25
Faci/o- root, 67
Fallopian tube, 123
FB (foreign body), 125
Femoral region, 25
Femor/o- root, 49
Fibr/o- root, 71
Flash cards, studying with, 5–6
Foley catheter, 123
Foramen/foramin- root, 71
Fore- prefix, 82
-form suffix, 111
Fossa root, 71
Fowler position, 21
Fowler's position, 123
Frank's sign, 123
Frontal plane, 21
Frontal region, 25
Fx (fracture/function), 131

G

Galact/o- root, 58, 71
Galactorrhea, vs. galacturia, 120

Galacturia, vs. galactorrhea, 120
Gangli/o- root, 52
Gastr/o- root, 44
-genesis suffix, 111
-genic suffix, 104
-gen suffix, 110
Ge pronunciation, 10
GERD (gastroesophageal reflux disease), 125
-geusia suffix, 111
Giga- prefix, 85
Gingiv/o- root, 67
Glauc/o- prefix, 86
Glomerul/o- root, 56
Gloss/o- prefix, 94
Gloss/o- root, 67
Gluc/o- root, 46
Gluteal region, 27
Glyc/o- root, 46
Gnath/o- root, 67
-gnosis suffix, 112
Gonad/o- root, 46
Gon/i- root, 71
Grammatical suffixes, 109–110
-gram suffix, 101
-graph suffix, 101
-graphy suffix, 101
Graves' disease, 124
Greek origins, 4, 11–13
Gtt (guttae), 127
Gues- root, 55
Gust/o- root, 55
Gynec/o- prefix, 92
Gynec/o- root, 58
Gyn/o- prefix, 92
Gyn/o- root, 58
Gyn pronunciation, 10

H

HAART (highly active antiretroviral therapy), 127
Hallus region, 25
Hb (hemoglobin), 131
HbA1c (glycated hemoglobin), 130
HD (hemodialysis), 129
Hecto- prefix, 85
Heimlich maneuver, 124
Hemat/o- root, 71
Hemi- prefix, 84
Hepat/o- root, 45
Hetero- prefix, 92
Hgb (hemoglobin), 131
Hidr/o- root, 47
Hippocrates, 11
Hist/o- root, 71
HIV (human immunodeficiency virus), 125
HLD (hyperlipidemia), 125
Hodgkin's lymphoma, 124
Homophones, 117, 118–122
Homo- prefix, 92
Horizontal plane, 20
HR (heart rate), 132
HRT (hormone replacement therapy), 129
HTN (hypertension), 126
Humeral, vs. humoral, 120
Humoral, vs. humeral, 120
Hydr/o- prefix, 88
Hydr/o- root, 71
Hyper- prefix, 88, 92
Hypochondriac region, 29
Hypogastric region, 30
Hypophysis, vs. hypothesis, 120
Hypo- prefix, 88, 92
Hypothenar region, 26
Hypothesis, vs. hypophysis, 120
Hyster/o- prefix, 94
Hyster/o- root, 58

I

-ial suffix, 110
-iasis suffix, 104
-ia suffix, 104
-iatrics suffix, 108
Iatr/o- prefix, 89
-iatry suffix, 108
IBD (inflammatory bowel disease), 126
IBS (irritable bowel syndrome), 126
Ichthy/o- root, 47
-ician suffix, 108
-ics suffix, 108
-ic suffix, 110
-ictal suffix, 104
ICU (intensive care unit), 129
Idio- prefix, 89
Ile/o- root, 45
Ileum, vs. ilium, 121
Iliac region, 27
Ilium, vs. ileum, 121
IM (intramuscular), 127
-ine suffix, 110
Inferior direction, 23, 73
Infra- prefix, 82
Inguinal region, 25
Inguin/o- root, 67
Integumentary system, 47–48
Internal direction, 23, 74
Inter- prefix, 82
Intra- prefix, 82
Intus- prefix, 82

-ion suffix, 112
Ipsi- prefix, 82
Irid/o- root, 55, 67
Ir/o- root, 55
Isch- prefix, 89
-ism suffix, 110
-ismus suffix, 104
Iso- prefix, 84
-ist suffix, 108
-itis suffix, 104
IUD (intrauterine device), 129
-ium suffix, 110
IV (intravenous), 127
IVF (IV fluids/in vitro
    fertilization), 129
IVP (intravenous push), 127

J

Jaund/o- prefix, 87
Jejun/o- root, 45

K

K (potassium), 127
Kal- root, 71
Kary- prefix, 89
Kerat/o- root, 48
Kilo- prefix, 85
Kine- root, 67
KVO (keep vein open), 129
Kyph/o- prefix, 82

L

Labi/a- root, 67
Labyrinth/o- root, 55
Lacrim/o- root, 55
Lact/o- root, 71

Lapar/o- root, 72
Laryng/o- root, 42
Lateral direction, 23, 74
Lateral recumbent/lateral decubitus
    position, 21
Later/o- prefix, 92
Latin origins, 4, 11–13
LBO (large bowel obstruction), 126
Left hypochondriac region, 30
Left iliac region, 30
Left lower quadrant (LLQ), 28
Left lumbar region, 30
Left upper quadrant (LUQ), 28
Lei/o- prefix, 89
Lept/o- prefix, 89
Leuk/o- prefix, 86
LFTs (liver function tests), 132
LGIB (lower gastrointestinal
    bleed), 126
Lice, vs. lyse, 121
Ling/o- prefix, 94
Ling/o- root, 67
Lingul/o- prefix, 94
Lingu/o- root, 67
Lip/o- root, 48
Lith/o- root, 57, 72
Lithotomy position, 22
-lith suffix, 104
-logist suffix, 108
-logy suffix, 108
Lord/o- prefix, 82
Lou Gehrig's disease, 124
LP (lumbar puncture), 129
Lumbar region, 24, 27, 31
Lyse, vs. lice, 121
-lysis suffix, 104
-lytic suffix, 105

M

Macro- prefix, 89
-malacia suffix, 105
Malleolus, vs. malleus, 121
Malleus, vs. malleolus, 121
Mal- prefix, 92, 94
Mammary region, 26
Mamm/o- prefix, 94
Mamm/o- root, 58, 67
-mania suffix, 105
MAP (mean arterial pressure), 132
Mast/o- prefix, 94
Mast/o- root, 59, 67
Measurement prefixes, 84–85
Medial direction, 23, 74
Median plane, 21
Medical terminology
  benefits of learning, 4–5
  components of, 4, 6–9
  defined, 4
  memorization tips, 5–6, 14–15
  origins of, 4, 11–13
  pluralizing, 13–14
  pronunciation of, 9–11
  quiz, 16
Medi/o- prefix, 92
-megaly suffix, 105
Mega- prefix, 85, 89
Melan/o- prefix, 86
Melanotic, vs. melenic, 121
Melenic, vs. melanotic, 121
Memorization tips, 5–6, 14–15, 80, 100
Mening/o- root, 53
Men/o- root, 59
mEq (milliequivalents), 127
Meso- prefix, 82
Metacarpal, vs. metatarsal, 121

Metaphysis, vs. metastasis, 121
Meta- prefix, 89
Metastasis, vs. metaphysis, 121
Metatarsal, vs. metacarpal, 121
-meter suffix, 101
Metric prefixes, 85
Metr/o- prefix, 94
Metr/o- root, 59
-metry suffix, 101
mg (milligrams), 127
MI (myocardial infarction), 126
Micro- prefix, 85, 89
Milli- prefix, 85
-mimetic suffix, 112
mL (milliliters), 127
Mohs surgery, 124
Mon/o- prefix, 84
-morph suffix, 112
MRI (mgnetic resonance
    imaging), 132
MS (multiple sclerosis), 126
Muscul/o- root, 49
Musculoskeletal system, 49–51
MVA (motor vehicle accident), 126
Myc/o- prefix, 89
Myel/o- root, 50, 53
My/o- root, 50
Myring/o- root, 55
Myx/o- prefix, 89

N

Na (sodium), 127
Nano- prefix, 85
Narc/o- prefix, 89
Nasal region, 25
Nas/o- prefix, 94
Nas/o- root, 42, 67

Nat/o- root, 72
Necr/o- prefix, 92
Necr/o- root, 72
Neo- prefix, 90
Nephr/o- prefix, 94
Nephr/o- root, 57
Nervous system, 52–53
Neur/o- root, 53
NG (nasogastric), 129
Nigr/o- prefix, 86
Noci/o- root, 53
Nodul/o- prefix, 90
Norm/o- prefix, 90
NPO (nil per os), 132
NS (normal saline), 128
NSAID (non-steroidal
    anti-inflammatory drug), 129
Nulli- prefix, 84
Number prefixes, 84–85
N/V (nausea and vomiting), 126

O

"o," use of in combining root
    words, 9, 39–40
Occipital region, 27
Occipit/o- root, 68
Ocular region, 25
Ocul/o- root, 55, 68
OD (oculus dexter), 132
Odont/o- prefix, 94
Odont/o- root, 68
Odyn/o- prefix, 90
-oid suffix, 110
Olfact/o- root, 55
Olig/o- prefix, 84
-ology suffix, 108
-ol suffix, 112

-oma suffix, 105
Omphal/o- prefix, 94
Omphal/o- root, 68
Onc/o- root, 72
Onych/o- prefix, 94
Onych/o- root, 48, 68
Oophor/o- prefix, 94
Oophor/o- root, 59
Ophthalm/o- root, 55, 68
-opia suffix, 108
Opposition, vs. apposition, 119
-opsy suffix, 101
Opt/o- root, 55, 68
Oral, vs. aural, 119
Oral region, 25
Orbital region, 25
Orchi/o- prefix, 94
Orchi/o- root, 60
Orch/o- prefix, 94
Orch/o- root, 60
Or/o- root, 45, 68
-orrhage/-orrhagia suffix, 105
Orth/o- prefix, 90
OS (oculus sinister), 132
OSA (obstructive sleep apnea), 126
-ose suffix, 112
-osis suffix, 110
Osmia root, 55
Osse/o- root, 50
Osteal, vs. ostial, 121
Oste/o- root, 50
Ostial, vs. osteal, 121
Ot/o- root, 55, 68
OU (oculus uterque), 132
-ous suffix, 110
Ovari/o- prefix, 94
Ovari/o- root, 59

Ov/o- root, 59
-oxia suffix, 105
Ox/i- root, 42
Oxy- prefix, 90

P

Pachy- prefix, 90
PAD (peripheral arterial
    disease), 126
Palmar direction, 23, 74
Palmar region, 26
Palpation, vs. palpitation, 121
Palpitation, vs. palpation, 121
Pancreat/o- root, 45
Pan- prefix, 90
Papill/o- root, 68
Para- prefix, 83
Parathyr/o- root, 46
-paresis suffix, 105
Parietal region, 27
Parkinson's disease, 124
Patellar region, 25
Patell/o- root, 50
Pathological condition
    suffixes, 103–107
Pathoma, 8
Path/o- prefix, 83
-pathy suffix, 105
Pauci- prefix, 84
PC (post cibum), 128
PE (pulmonary embolism), 126
PEA (pulseless electrical
    activity), 126
Pectoral region, 26
Pector- root, 68
Pedal region, 25

PEG (percutaneous gastrostomy
    tube), 130
Pelvic cavity, 32
Pelv/o- root, 68
-penia suffix, 105
-pepsia suffix, 108
Perfuse, vs. profuse, 122
Perineal, vs. peroneal, 121
Perineal region, 27
Perine/o- root, 68
Peri- prefix, 83
Peroneal, vs. perineal, 121
Per- prefix, 83
-pexy suffix, 102
-phagia/-phago/-phagy suffix, 105
Phalangeal region, 26
Phall/o- root, 60, 69
Pharmaceutical abbreviations,
    127–128
Pharmaco- prefix, 90
Pharyng/o- root, 45
-phasia suffix, 105
-pheresis suffix, 102
-phil/-philic suffix, 112
Phleb/o- root, 41
Phleb- prefix, 94
-phobia suffix, 105
-phonia suffix, 106
Phon/o- root, 55
-phoria suffix, 106
Phos- root, 72
Phot/o- root, 56
Ph pronunciation, 10
Phren/o- root, 42
-physis suffix, 112
Pico- prefix, 85
Pil/o- prefix, 94

Pil/o- root, 48, 69
Pituitar/o- root, 47
Plantar direction, 23, 74
Plantar region, 27
-plasia suffix, 112
-plasm suffix, 112
-plasty suffix, 102
-plegia suffix, 106
Pleio- prefix, 84
Pleural, vs. plural, 121
Pleur/o- root, 43
-plexy suffix, 106
PLT (platelets), 132
Plural, vs. pleural, 121
Pluralizing terms, 13–14
-pnea suffix, 108
Pneum/o- root, 43
Pn pronunciation, 10
PO (per os), 128
Pod/o- root, 50, 69
-poeisis suffix, 112
Poly- prefix, 84
Popliteal region, 27
-porosis suffix, 106
Positions, body, 21–22, 80–83
Posterior direction, 23, 74
Poster/o- prefix, 92
Post- prefix, 83
PPI (proton pump inhibitor), 130
PR (per rectum), 128
-prandial suffix, 113
Prefixes
  about, 7, 79, 95
  antonyms, 92–93
  color, 86–87
  combining root words with, 75

common, 87–91
memorization tips, 80
metric, 85
number and measurement, 84–85
position and direction, 80–83
quiz, 96
synonyms, 94
Pre- prefix, 83
Presby- root, 72
Prim/i- prefix, 84
PRN (pro re nata), 128
Procine- prefix, 90
Proct/o- root, 45
Professional suffixes, 107–109
Profuse, vs. perfuse, 122
Prone position, 22
Pronunciation tips, 9–11
Pro- prefix, 83
Prostate, vs. prostrate, 122
Prostat/o- root, 60
Prostrate, vs. prostate, 122
Proximal direction, 23, 74
Pseud/o- prefix, 90
Ps pronunciation, 10
Psych/o- root, 53
PT (physical therapy), 130
Pter pronunciation, 10
-ptosis suffix, 106
-ptysis suffix, 106
Pubic region, 25
Purpur/o- prefix, 86
PVD (peripheral vascular
  disease), 126
Pyel/o- root, 57
Py/o- prefix, 90
Pyr/o- root, 72

Q

Q2h/Q3h/Q4h (every two, three, or four hours), 128
QAM (every morning), 128
QD (quaque die), 128
QHS (quaque hora somni), 128
QID (quater in die), 128
QPM (every evening), 128
Quadrants, abdominal, 28
Quadri- prefix, 85
Quizzes
  body, 34
  medical terminology overview, 16
  prefixes, 96
  root words, 62–63, 77
  suffixes, 115

R

RA (room air), 132
Radicul/o- root, 53
RBC (red blood cells), 132
Rect/o- root, 45
Regions
  abdominal-pelvic, 29–30
  anterior, 25–26
  posterior, 27
  spinal, 24, 31
Ren/o- prefix, 94
Ren/o- root, 57
Re- prefix, 90
Reproductive system
  female, 58–59
  male, 60
Respiratory system, 42–43
Reticul/o- prefix, 91
Retr/o- prefix, 92

Retro- prefix, 83
Reverse Trendelenburg position, 22
Rheu pronunciation, 10
Rhin/o- prefix, 94
Rhin/o- root, 43, 69
Right hypochondriac region, 29
Right iliac region, 29
Right lower quadrant (RLQ), 28
Right lumbar region, 29
Right upper quadrant (RUQ), 28
ROM (range of motion), 132
Root words
  about, 7, 39–40, 61, 76
  cardiovascular system, 40–41
  combining with suffixes and
    prefixes, 75
  digestive system, 44–45
  directional, 73–75
  endocrine system, 46–47
  external body parts, 66–69
  integumentary system, 47–48
  internal body parts, 70–72
  musculoskeletal system, 49–51
  nervous system, 52–53
  quiz, 62–63, 77
  reproductive system, female, 58–59
  reproductive system, male, 60
  respiratory system, 42–43
  sensory system, 54–56
  urinary system, 56–57
-rrhaphy suffix, 102
-rrhea suffix, 106
-rrhexis suffix, 106
RRT (rapid response team), 130
RT (respiratory therapy), 130
Rubr/o- prefix, 86

S

s/ (without), 132
Sacral region, 24, 27, 31
Sagittal plane, 21
Salping/o- root, 59
Sanguin- prefix, 91
-sarcoma suffix, 106
Sarc/o- root, 50
SBO (small bowel obstruction), 126
SBP (systolic blood pressure), 132
Scapular region, 27
-schisis suffix, 107
-sclerosis suffix, 107
Scoli/o- prefix, 91
-scope suffix, 102
-scopic suffix, 102
-scopy suffix, 102
Scrot/o- root, 60
SC/subQ (subcutaneous), 128
Seb/o- root, 48
Semi- prefix, 85
Sensory system, 54–56
-sepsis suffix, 107
Sept/o- root, 72
Ser/o- root, 72
Sial/o- root, 45
Sigmoid/o- root, 45
Sinistr/o- prefix, 83
Sinus/o- root, 43
SNF (skilled nursing facility), 132
SOB (shortness of breath), 132
Somat/o- prefix, 91
Somat/o- root, 69
Somn/o- root, 53
-spadias suffix, 107
-spasm suffix, 107
Specialty suffixes, 107–109

Spinal cavity/canal, 32
Spinal regions, 24, 31
Spin/o- root, 53
Spir/o- root, 43
Splen/o- root, 45
Spondyl/o- root, 50
Squamos/o- root, 48
-stalsis suffix, 113
-stasis suffix, 113
STAT (statium), 128
-stenosis suffix, 113
Sternal region, 26
Stern/o- root, 50
Steth/o- root, 69
Stomat/o- prefix, 91
Stomat/o- root, 69
-stomy suffix, 102
Sub- prefix, 83
Subxiphoid region, 26
Suffixes
  about, 7–8, 99, 114
  combining root words with, 75
  common, 111–113
  grammatical, 109–110
  memorization tips, 100
  pathological conditions, 103–107
  professionals and
    specialties, 107–109
  quiz, 115
  surgical and diagnostic, 100–102
Superficial direction, 23, 74
Superior direction, 23, 73
Super/supra- prefix, 83
Supine position, 21
Sural region, 27
Surgical suffixes, 100–102
Symbols, 133

Synonyms, 94
Syn/o- root, 50
Syn/sym- prefix, 91
Systol/e- root, 41

T

T (temperature), 132
Tab (tablet), 128
Tachy- prefix, 91, 92
TAH (total abdominal
    hysterectomy), 130
Tal/o- root, 50, 69
Tarsal region, 26, 27
Tars/o- root, 51, 69
TAVR (transcatheter aortic valve
    replacement), 130
Temporal region, 25
Ten/o- root, 51
Tension root, 41
-tension/-tensive suffix, 113
Tera- prefix, 85
Terat/o- root, 72
Testicul/o- prefix, 94
Test/o- prefix, 94
Test/o- root, 60
Tetan/o- root, 72
Tetra- prefix, 85
THA (total hip arthroplasty), 130
Thenar region, 26
Therm/o- root, 72
Thoracic cavity, 24, 32
Thoracic region, 24, 26, 31
Thorac/o- root, 69
-thorax suffix, 109
Thromb/o- root, 72
Thym/o- root, 53
Thyroid/o- root, 47

-tic suffix, 110
TID (ter in die), 128
-tion suffix, 113
TKA (total knee arthroplasty), 130
-tome suffix, 102
Tommy John surgery, 124
Tort/o- root, 51
-toxic suffix, 113
TPN (total parenteral nutrition), 128
Trache/o- root, 43, 69
Track, vs. tract, 122
Tract, vs. track, 122
Trans- prefix, 83, 91, 92
Transverse plane, 20
Trendelenburg position, 22
Trich/o- prefix, 94
Trich/o- root, 48, 69
Tri- prefix, 85
-tripsy suffix, 102
-trophy suffix, 113
Tympan/o- root, 56

U

UA (urinalysis), 132
UGIB (upper gastrointestinal
    bleed), 126
-ula/-ule suffix, 110
Ultra- prefix, 91
Umbilical region, 25, 30
Umbilic/o- prefix, 94
Ungu/o- prefix, 94
Ungu/o- root, 48
Uni- prefix, 85
Ureter/o- root, 57
Urethr/o- root, 57
-uria suffix, 109
Urinary system, 56–57

Urin/o- root, 57
Ur/o- roo, 57
Uter/o- prefix, 94
Uter/o- root, 59
UTI (urinary tract infection), 126
Uve/o- root, 56

V

Vagin/o- prefix, 94
Vagin/o- root, 59
Valgus direction, 74
Valv/o- root, 41
Valvul/o- root, 41
Varus direction, 75
Vascul/o- root, 41
Vas/o- root, 41
VBG (venous blood gas), 132
Vein/o- prefix, 94
Ven/o- root, 41
Ventral cavity, 32
Ventral direction, 73
Ventricul/o- root, 41
Vertebral region, 27
Vertebr/o- root, 51

Vesical, vs. vesicle, 122
Vesicle, vs. vesical, 122
Vesic/o- root, 57
VF (ventricular fibrillation), 126
Viscous, vs. viscus, 122
Viscus, vs. viscous, 122
VT (ventricular tachycardia), 126
Vulv/o- root, 59

W

w/ (with), 132
WBC (white blood cells), 132
w/o (without), 132

X

Xanth/o- prefix, 87
Xeno- prefix, 91
Xer/o- prefix, 91
Xero pronunciation, 10

Y

YO (years old), 132
-y suffix, 113

ACKNOWLEDGMENTS

I want to thank you for purchasing this book and for putting in the time and effort to learn the medical language. I hope you will remember how you felt at the start of this journey, before learning medical terminology. As you grow your medical knowledge, please try to empathize with those around you who have little or no exposure to these terms and do your best to translate medical terms in a way they can understand. This will help us all better communicate and connect.

I want to thank all my teachers: my professors, colleagues, interns, residents, and students. You have all added to my knowledge. Most of all, I want to thank my patients, who have been my ultimate teachers. Nothing we learn in medicine is ever as memorable as it becomes when we connect it with a patient. It is truly an honor to learn from, with, and about you.

ABOUT THE AUTHOR

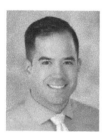 **John Louis Temple, MD,** is an internal medicine–trained academic hospitalist physician and former chief resident who practices in Southern California. His academic interests include quality improvement, patient safety, patient experience, and medical education. When he is not at work, he spends his time surfing, gardening, composting, and hanging out with his family.